Created
&Called

A Journey to and through Nursing

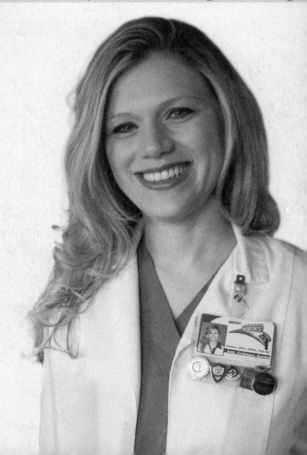

CHELSIA HARRIS,
DNP, APRN, FNP-BC

First printing: August 2015

New Leaf Press, P.O. Box 726, Green Forest, AR 72638

New Leaf Press is a division of the New Leaf Publishing Group, Inc.

ISBN: 978-0-89221-736-6
Library of Congress Number: 2015946959

Cover by Diana Bogardus

Unless otherwise noted, Scripture quotations are from the English Standard Version (ESV) of the Bible.

Please consider requesting that a copy of this volume be purchased by your local library system.

Printed in the United States of America

Please visit our website for other great titles:
www.newleafpress.net

For information regarding author interviews, please contact the publicity department at (870) 438-5288.

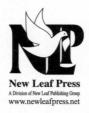

New Leaf Press
A Division of New Leaf Publishing Group
www.newleafpress.net

Contents

1 . The Call 5

2 . The Purpose of a Nurse 15

3 . It's All about the Blood 21

4 . A Legacy of Light 27

5 . Compassionate Care 33

6 . Sacrificial Service 41

7 . Humble Heart, Helping Hands 49

8 . Integrity Is Integral 55

9 . Communication and Collaboration: Critical Care 63

10 . Organization Is Not Optional 71

11 . A Firm Foundation: Curriculum Choices 79

12 . The Temperature of Nursing: A Range of Degrees 87

13 . Endless Opportunities 93

14 . It's More than Salary 99

15 . Nursing Process: Just AD-PIE 105

16 . Sights, Sounds, Smells . . . Oh My! 111

17 . Death and Dying: A Heavy Heart 115

18 . Mind, Body, Spirit: Triune Care 123

19 . Creating a Nourishing Environment 129

20 . Patients Require Patience 137

21 . Fatigued but Not Finished: A Prescription
       for Perseverance 143

22 . Memorable Moments 149

23 . Answering the Call 161

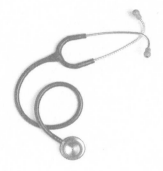

Chapter 1

The Call

Have you ever wondered, "What are my gifts? What exactly is God calling me to do with my life?" It was 1999 and I was assisting my 83-year-old great-aunt Mart with a bath, when she asked me, "Have you ever thought about working with the 'old people'?" I pondered for a moment. That was a question I had to think about to answer. Now, I have to tell you that my Aunt Mart was a woman of impeccable, godly character. I never met my maternal grandmother. She died long before I was born. So her sister, Aunt Mart, filled the shoes of the grandma role in my life. Aunt Mart never had children of her own, never drove a day in her life, was widowed in 1986, and depended solely upon the Lord to meet her needs. Although Aunt Mart never had her own biological children, she had many children. I cannot remember a single weekend we didn't visit my Aunt Mart and climb the trees in her front yard with all of my cousins. After everyone would leave, I would go inside, crawl up in Aunt Mart's lap, and run my fingers across the velvety soft, wrinkled skin of her hand. She would caress my hair and tell me how beautiful she thought I was and how I must always "serve the Lord and lay every burden at His feet."

Aunt Mart fixed the best chicken strips and sugary frozen strawberries. She loved me and my brother and cousins more than anything. She never forgot a birthday and you could bank on it, at Christmas, every single one of our family members would cram ourselves into Aunt Mart's little humble home to celebrate the birth of Jesus Christ. Aunt Mart didn't have much, but she had plenty. Her house smelled of coffee and the vapors of her water cooler in the summer, and her wood burning stove in the winter. I loved my Aunt Mart!

In the year 2000, I graduated from Atkins High School in Atkins, Arkansas. There were only 68 students in my class. My Aunt Mart was so proud! By this time, she had such a severe curvature in her spine that her chin almost touched her waist

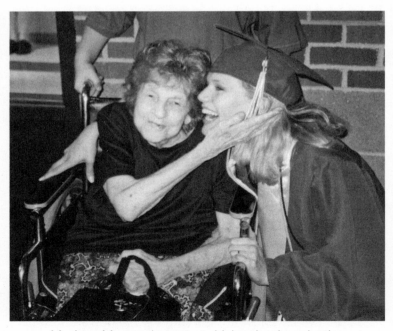

My Aunt Mart and me at my high school graduation

when she stood. You see, osteoporosis had weakened her bones immensely. As a young woman, Aunt Mart was 5 feet 6 inches tall, but on the day of my high school graduation, she stood only 4 feet 11 inches. She really wasn't able to stand too much. She had to be wheeled into the auditorium in her wheelchair. However, Aunt Mart wouldn't have missed that day for the world! Aunt Mart was often in tremendous amounts of pain, but you would have never known it. She didn't complain about anything. She felt as if each day was a gift from the Lord and that we should "rejoice and be glad in it."

I was rejoicing that particular night! Graduation night. May 10, 2000. I walked across that stage to receive my diploma with Aunt Mart's question, "Have you ever thought about working with the 'old people'?" resonating in my heart and mind. I hadn't necessarily felt that I would work with the "old people," but I knew that God was calling me to a life of service. I had already registered for college and declared nursing as my major. My plan was to get my Bachelor of Science in Nursing (BSN) degree and work the rest of my life on a pediatric oncology unit. What I didn't know at the young age of 17 was that "the heart of man plans his way, but the LORD establishes his steps" (Proverbs 16:9).

Spring break of my sophomore year of college, I received the phone call. This call was one that brought me to my knees. It was my uncle. He said, "Aunt Mart has fallen, and it's pretty bad." My cousin found her 45 minutes after her fall, lying in a pool of blood in her living room. Aunt Mart was independent. She didn't allow many people to wait on her. That particular day, she was adjusting the heat on her stove. It was still cold in Arkansas at this time. When she turned around she lost her balance, fell backwards, and hit her head on the concrete cinder blocks that she used for book shelves.

I cried as my uncle explained the situation that Aunt Mart was in trouble and was being transported to the hospital. Since I was out of state when I received the call, it took me 48 hours to get to Aunt Mart. When I walked into her room, my heart sank! The smell almost knocked me down, and the sight was horrific! Aunt Mart's sheets, pillow, face, and head were covered in dried blood. She had not even had so much as a warm, moist cloth rubbed across her face. Where were the nurses?!? Had they forgotten about my precious aunt? Was she not worthy of quality care? Again, Aunt Mart's question resonated loudly in my heart and mind: "Have you ever thought about working with the 'old people'?" At that very moment, I wanted to shout to the rooftop, "YES, Aunt Mart, YES!" But she was sedated and couldn't respond to me.

Days went by as my family remained close to Aunt Mart's hospital bed. We clung to every moment. We would gather around her bed and pray or sing hymns. We took turns sleeping overnight in her room. There was never one minute of any day that there were not at least four or five of us there. Minute by minute, I watched in disbelief as my Aunt Mart struggled to hang on to life. My heart broke when she would scream out in horrific pain. The doctors informed us that the pain was because Aunt Mart had fractured almost every vertebra in her spine, secondary to the osteoporosis and fall. I just wanted to comfort her. I wanted to take her pain away. In those moments, I wanted to be her nurse.

The tables had turned. It was now me caressing Aunt Mart's hair, telling her how beautiful she was, and how I was trying so desperately to lay my burdens at Jesus' feet. As Aunt Mart was taking her final breaths, I felt the call to nursing stronger than I ever had before. My heart began to beat wildly in my chest, and I felt as if it might stop along with Aunt Mart's. My lungs felt like a balloon that someone had just stuck with a pin. The air was slowly leaking out, but there was nothing coming back in to replace it. Goose bumps covered my body. My hands trembled. The woman I had loved, admired, and revered as the closest thing to Jesus I had ever known was slipping away, and I couldn't stop it.

One last time, I ran my trembling fingers over the velvety soft, wrinkled skin of Aunt Mart's hand. "Thank you. I love you," I whispered. In that moment, I realized that God had used my sweet Aunt Mart to "call" me to be a nurse. I vowed to spend the rest of my life ensuring that every patient, young or old, was valued and received compassionate, high-quality care. I wasn't exactly sure how I would fulfill that promise, but I felt deep in my spirit that God was going to equip me.

Two years later, I was lying in bed tossing and turning as I thought of the exam I would take the next morning — the most exciting, dreaded, and important examination of my life. The exam that would tell me whether I would be able to obtain my Registered Nursing (RN) license — the standardized National Council (of State Boards of Nursing) Licensure Exam for Registered Nurses (NCLEX – RN).

Through the pounding of my heart and the racing of my mind, I heard a still, small voice telling me that I was going to pass. I felt an intense peace and calm come over my body. The Holy Spirit was with me. As my heartbeat slowed, I began to think of my Aunt Mart. Tomorrow I would take that test for her. I would take that test for all of the people that needed a nurse that truly cared. I would take that test to fulfill the calling that God had placed upon my life. As I drifted off to sleep, I am convinced that I felt that velvety soft, wrinkled hand holding mine once again.

The next morning, I passed the test! So, the journey began. The first two years, I worked on a medical-surgical floor in a small community hospital in Branson, Missouri. The majority of my patients were greater than age 65. Many people felt the night shift would be difficult and that I might burn out easily.

However, I loved the night shift, but more than that, I just loved being a nurse! The fulfillment I got from helping ease someone's pain or from comforting a family member after the loss of their loved one was inexplicable! Often times, when the other nurses couldn't find me, they joked that all they had to do was follow the talking and laughter into one of my patient's rooms. This was a season in my life that I will cherish forever.

However, this season didn't last long. After two years of working as a nurse at the bedside, I began to feel that yearning in my spirit, that still, small voice, telling me that God was calling me, yet again, to something more, something bigger. I was reminded of the Scripture: "For everything there is a season, and a time for every matter under heaven" (Ecclesiastes 3:1). This was a season of my life, but the season was about to change.

In 2008, I finished my Masters of Science in Nursing (MSN) degree! After passing a national certification exam, I was officially a Family Nurse Practitioner! Being a nurse in the hospital receiving orders from the doctors was one thing; writing the orders and managing patient care by myself was

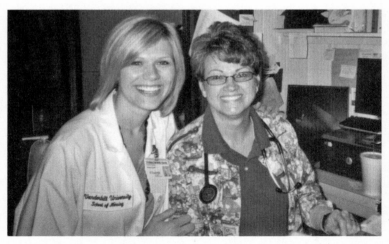

Linda McIntosh (Family Nurse Practitioner Preceptor) and me

completely different. I was scared to death! The Lord comforted me by reminding me that He "gave us a spirit not of fear but of power and love and self-control" (2 Timothy 1:7). Over the next several months, my fear lessened. I thoroughly enjoyed having my own patients and caring for their physical, emotional, and spiritual needs. I loved my job and being a nurse practitioner. I thought this was going to be the job I did for the rest of my life. I was wrong again!

Fortunately, God's plan is far better than our plans. One day as I sat at my desk answering emails and finishing patient charts, my phone rang. I answered. It was the director of a BSN program at a private Christian college in southern Missouri. She was inquiring about using our facility as a clinical site. After several minutes of conversation, she said that their program was looking for an additional nursing professor. I immediately stated that I was not interested; teenagers and young adults were not who God had called me to serve, and I had never taught a day in my life. The woman simply said, "Would you pray about it?" Oh, no! Pray about it. How could she ask me such a thing?! "Sure," I said hesitantly. We hung up the phone and I went about my business.

For weeks, I, halfheartedly, prayed about the request. Every day I would feel the Lord tugging at my heartstrings. "This cannot be what You have called me to do, Lord. You want me to be a nurse, not a teacher. I promised my Aunt Mart and You that I would spend my life ensuring that Your children, my patients, would receive compassionate, high-quality care. I love my patients. I am a good nurse. I could never be a teacher. I don't even know how to speak in front of people. Please don't make me do this," I pleaded with the Lord. He did not reply in an audible voice, but I knew things were about to change.

Over the next several weeks, things began to happen that some people would call coincidental, but I knew were divine.

On one occasion, I received a phone call from a college professor in Arkansas. She asked me if I would come and speak to their freshmen about the nursing profession. The woman said that I had come "highly recommended." Highly recommended? The only time I had ever spoken in front of an audience was years ago in pageants nowhere near this town. How could I have been "highly recommended"? Then, there was that still, small voice again, "Go, I will equip you." I asked the lady what day and time she would like me to be there.

Speaking to that class was invigorating! I shared my story and expressed the passion and compassion it takes to be a nurse. One young lady even told me that I should be a teacher because I was a "great speaker." Was God using these people as vessels to speak into my life? To help me better understand my gifts? To make me realize my calling? Was He really asking me to be a teacher? Several more inexplicable, divine appointments ensued. I often argued with the Lord that, if I became a nursing professor, I would no longer be able to take care of His people and fulfill the calling He had placed on my life. Then I realized that, if I became a nursing professor, I would be training more nurses to go out into the world and serve patients with kindness, love, and compassion. My circle of influence would be multiplied immensely. Every nurse that I helped to train would serve their patients and then, if they became educators, the nurses that they trained would serve their patients, and so on and so on. This vision excited me!

The excitement continues today. I took that job as a nursing professor six years ago. Since the first day I stepped foot onto the college campus at College of the Ozarks in Point Lookout, Missouri, I feel as if I have been hovering off of the ground. Every day, I float into work with a smile on my face and joy in my heart. I teach young men and women what it means to be a nurse and how to be a godly nurse full of love and compassion. A picture of my Aunt Mart remains in my office as a daily reminder of how God used a woman of small stature to call me to great things much bigger than anything I could have ever imagined.

So now, I ask you again, have you ever wondered, "What are my gifts? What exactly is God calling me to do with my life?" I can probably safely assume that you have asked yourself these questions, and since you are reading this book, you may have pondered the idea of becoming a nurse. I challenge you to keep your heart and mind open. Your plans may be different from the plans that God has for your life. You may be telling yourself that you do not have the ability to be a nurse or speak in front of large crowds or write a book. Believe me, I said those things too. But we can do all things through Christ who strengthens us (Philippians 4:13). It is my prayer that, as you read this book, you will search your heart, cultivate a deeper, more intimate relationship with Jesus Christ, and close the book knowing whether God is calling you to this incredible, humbling profession called nursing.

My Prayer for You

Heavenly Father,

You are the God of all creation. Lord over heaven and all the earth. You are the Alpha and Omega. The Beginning and the End. Your love for Your children is unconditional. You knit each one of us together in our mothers' wombs. We were fearfully and wonderfully made. You have given each one of us gifts — gifts that are to be used for Your glory, to further Your Kingdom. Father, I ask that You bless the person reading this book. I ask that You penetrate their heart. Send Your Holy Spirit to encourage and comfort them. Give them a spirit of discernment. Help them to know what it is that

You are calling them to do. If You are calling them to the nursing profession, instill a passion so deep and so wide within their souls that they do not question Your plan. May the world stand at attention, curious to know from where the light that shines from within them is coming. Lord, bless them beyond measure. I thank You for them. I praise You for the gifts that You have given them. Continue to cultivate those gifts and allow them to share these gifts with others.

In Jesus' Holy and most precious name, Amen.

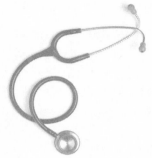

Chapter 2

The Purpose of a Nurse

Purpose. The reason why something is done. "The Lord has made everything for its purpose" (Proverbs 16:4). The purpose of a nurse is multifaceted. A nurse is a helper, a servant, a leader, an advocate, an educator, a comforter, an encourager, a prayer warrior, and a team player. But how can one person be so many things?

Picture this. You are a nurse in the emergency department. It has been a hectic day. It is only noon, and you have already taken care of a man with crushing chest pain, a woman with uncontrolled seizures, a child with a fever of an unknown origin, a teenager involved in a motorcycle accident, and you just finished washing the feet of a homeless man with countless diabetic ulcers covering the surface of both of his feet and legs. You have not gotten the chance to sit down for the last five hours. However, the chaos has recently come to a lull. All of your patients are settled and you are just about to sit down to document in your last patient's chart. Your back aches and your mind is exhausted. You plop down into the rolling desk chair to finish your charting. It feels like a Lazy boy recliner at this point. You roll the chair under the desk and place your fingers on the keyboard to sign into the computer.

Suddenly, all you hear are blood-curdling screams. It's a mother flying frantically through the sliding glass doors of the emergency room. She's holding her blue, lifeless baby boy, screaming, "SOMEONE HELP ME, PLEASE! HELP MY BABY!" You instantaneously forget about your aching back and exhausted mind. Adrenaline is pumping through your veins. It is almost as if you have received supernatural energy. You race to the mother's side and introduce yourself as the nurse. The mother looks into your eyes yearning for reassurance. You take the baby, cradle him in your arms, and quickly escort them to a private room.

You lay the baby down onto the exam table. You get onto the table next to the baby and place the palm of your hand in the center of his chest. Before you have even had a chance to think, you have already begun chest compressions. You delegate to the patient care technician to remain with the mother and comfort her while the rest of the healthcare team takes care of the baby. You lead cardiopulmonary resuscitation (CPR) until the doctor and respiratory therapist arrive. While continuing chest compressions, gathering a health history on the baby, encouraging and comforting the mother with reassuring eye contact and an occasional nod, you are also silently pleading with the Lord to give you wisdom and to save this baby's life.

Just as you are pressing one last time on the chest of the lifeless baby, you look down. You see color flooding into his cheeks. The scream coming from his mouth is the most beautiful noise that you have ever heard. "He is breathing! Thank you, Jesus! He is breathing!" you whisper quietly. Your heart quickens as you remember Scripture. "Then the LORD God formed the man of dust from the ground and breathed into his nostrils the breath of life, and the man became a living creature" (Genesis 2:7). The Lord had just breathed the breath of life back into this baby!

The mother, still sobbing, rushes over and embraces you from behind, almost pulling you off of the exam table onto the floor. She is holding you so tightly that you can barely breathe yourself. You hop off of the exam table, turn to face her, and envelop her in your arms. You can feel her heart pounding against your chest. Your heart is beating equally as hard. It is almost as if your hearts are beating in sync with one another. As you are entwined in the embrace, you silently thank God for that mother and baby and ask Him to protect them and to bless them beyond measure. In a matter of a single morning, you, the nurse, were a helper, a servant, a leader, a comforter, an encourager, a team player, and a prayer warrior.

Thirty minutes later, all is calm and the baby is resting quietly. At this time, you offer the mother your undivided attention as she struggles to tell you what happened. She informs you that her baby is 18 months old and that he is her first and only child. She explains that she got pregnant out of wedlock at age 16, the daddy is no longer in the picture, her parents have disowned her, and she is struggling to make ends meet. In reality, she is still just a child herself. She puts her face in her hands and begins crying again. She tells you that she is to blame for all of this. You sit quietly and listen as she continues to explain the details of that frightening morning.

The baby was sitting in his high chair in the kitchen, eating dry cereal. Through sobs, she tells you that she was folding a load of laundry and putting on the final touches of her makeup in the next room. You hand her a tissue and place your hand on her arm. She continues to explain that, since she is the sole provider for her family, she has to work. She blots her eyes with the tissue. You notice her hands are trembling. She looks up at you and says, "I was just trying to finish getting ready for work before I had to drop my baby off at daycare. I cannot believe that I am so stupid!" she says through gritted teeth. "This is all so hard. I'm a horrible mother! I don't think I can continue to do this!" You help ease her down into a chair, pull up a chair next to her, and turn your body to face her. As you look into her teary-blue eyes, you can see the years of pain and anguish. Your heart aches for her. In the most tender and convincing way possible, you reassure her that you are there to help.

You see the furrow in her brow soften, and the tremor in her hands begins to decrease. She trusts you. She takes a deep breath and continues the story. "Several minutes had passed and I didn't hear my baby. He is usually jabbering and banging his hands on the high chair tray. So I ran into the kitchen, and that's when I saw him." She fights back tears again. "My baby was slumped forward in his highchair. He was not breathing and his skin was grayish blue." You nod to assure her that you are still listening. "I immediately grabbed him out of the high-chair and pounded on his back. Nothing happened. His eyes were rolled back in his head. His lips were blue. I was so scared! I thought he was dead! All I could think about was how my mother and father were right. I am worthless! I will never be good mother!"

As the nurse, you know that your job was not finished when you completed the final chest compression. Your purpose continues now as you take on the role of comforter, educator, and advocate. You again place your hand on the mother's arm and assure her that you are not there to judge her or point fingers as you remember the Scripture: "Judgment is without mercy to one who has shown no mercy. Mercy triumphs over judgment" (James 2:13). Her gaze looks up from the floor back into your eyes. You can see a glimmer of hope within her. You explain to her that you are going to contact the chaplain to come in and visit with her and to provide emotional and spiritual support.

You also tell her that you will contact social services to help her explore various resources available for single mothers. Her lips form a smile. She lunges forward, embracing you like a child that has just been reunited with her mother. She thanks you over and over again. Your heart swells and you offer a quiet, "You're welcome."

As you wrap up the conversation, you express to the mother the importance of knowing how to protect her child if another incident occurs in the future. She agrees. You enroll her in the basic first aid and CPR course in your hospital. You know that this education will empower her and provide her with a sense of peace. At that moment, the doctor comes in and informs the mother that her baby is doing great and she is free to go. You assist the mother in gathering her things, and hand her all of the discharge information and contact phone numbers that she may need in the future. She cradles her baby in her arms. You wave goodbye as the mother and her baby walk slowly through the hospital doors and venture back out into the world. You wonder if you did enough. You pray for God's purpose to be completed in their lives. Then you turn around and walk down the hallway to provide the same quality of care to the next patient awaiting you.

Hopefully, through this story, you have recognized that the purpose of a nurse runs deep. Nurses are more than crisp, clean uniforms and shiny, white shoes. We offer help and service to those in need. We humbly and respectfully lead the care of our patients. We advocate for quality healthcare. We educate to empower. We comfort the brokenhearted. We encourage the lowly in spirit. We pray without ceasing. We are valuable members of the healthcare team. We are fulfilling God's purposeful call to nursing!

My Prayer for You

Heavenly Father,

Thank You for creating us and giving us the breath of life. Without You, we are nothing. We have no purpose but, in You, we find our purpose and can do all things. Thank You for loving us so much that You would allow us to be vessels to fulfill Your purpose. I pray that the person reading this book will cry out to You, the Most High God, so that You may fulfill Your purpose in them. Lord, if it is Your plan for them to become a nurse, I pray that You will instill in them a deep desire to help, serve, lead, advocate, educate, comfort, encourage, and pray for Your children as they participate as members of the healthcare team and the Body of Christ. I love You, Lord, and I give You all the praise!

In Jesus' Holy and most precious name, Amen.

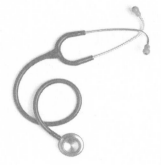

Chapter 3

It's All about
the Blood

Throughout my career, I have met many people. People of great character with high moral and ethical standards. People with kind, loving, compassionate, servant's hearts. People who would make incredible nurses! These people frequently express to me their desire to help others through the profession of nursing. They speak with passion fueling their words. However, sadly, before they even embark on the adventure to nursing, they abruptly close the door because they are fearful or become ill at the sight of blood. I pray that some of these passionate people are reading this book and that this chapter changes their lives!

Think about a river. A river begins at a source and travels through a channel created by riverbanks on either side. The water in a river continuously flows, unless a human or animal builds a dam and hinders it. Rivers are full of life. Many fish, turtles, and reptiles call a river home. Rivers supply larger animals and humans with a food and water source to provide nourishment. The roots of trees and plants along the banks run deep to have access to the river water. The banks of a river swell with the rains and recede with the sun. Rivers carry barges and ships across the world to distribute goods and services. Rivers produce electricity. Rivers offer beauty for the human eyes to indulge. Rivers can be a place of fun for families to create memories from camping, fishing, and rafting. Rivers do not freeze in the bitter cold, and they rarely dry up in the heat. Rivers are an incredible creation!

Blood is the river of life! Ninety percent of blood is comprised of water. And, much like the water in a river, blood flows. The source of blood is the bone marrow, where red blood cells are produced. The channels and riverbanks for blood are the arteries and veins. Blood is continuously flowing. Vessels constrict and dilate with various activities, medications, and disease processes, increasing or decreasing the pressure and velocity with which blood flows. If humans consume too much fat in their diet, the fat can form deposits that act like tiny dams in the vessels and hinder the flow of blood.

Blood is home to many life-sustaining elements. Blood carries red blood cells that carry oxygen. Oxygen is necessary for life. Blood travels through the heart. Arteries carry the blood to the lungs to be oxygenated. There, the oxygenated blood is pumped back out into the body. It travels from very large vessels over hills and valleys, much like a river. The large vessels supply the brain and other vital organs with blood and nutrients. Then the blood continues to push itself onward into extremely tiny capillaries. Capillaries supply body parts such as the hands, fingers, feet, toes, ears, and nose with blood. Then blood travels back to the heart through veins. Muscles help force the blood back to the heart through gates and passageways called valves to start the whole process over again.

White blood cells are also carried by the blood. White blood cells are vital to our immune system functionality. When inflammation or infection plagues our bodies, the amount of white blood cells increases to cleanse the body of the unwanted material. Platelets, plasma, and proteins are also carried by the blood, and if the blood ceased to carry them, we would surely die. Blood also regulates the acid/base balance in our bodies and keeps us in a homeostatic state. Blood warms us when we are too cold and cools us when we are too hot. So think about the importance and the value of blood.

Pretend you are the nurse in a small, private nursing home. You have worked there for seven years. You try not too get attached to the residents because you know that this is their last destination before heaven, and your heart just cannot bear the burden of loss. However, five years ago a young woman pushed her father in a wheelchair through the front doors of the nursing home, turned around, walked out, and never returned.

Upon arrival, you discovered that the new resident was 96 years old. His skin was wrinkled and leathery from the years he worked as a farmer, not to mention the time he spent as a sailor in the United States Navy protecting your freedom. This man intrigued you. You logged hours listening to stories of Pearl Harbor, Normandy, and his love of his country. He explained to you that he had become a burden on his family since his stroke. He could no longer walk, was confined to a wheelchair, and often required assistance with his activities of daily living, such as brushing his teeth, showering, and eating. Previously, you considered assisting with such things to be a chore. However, with this gentleman, it was different. You felt it was your honor and privilege to serve him. After all, he risked his life for your freedom.

Days, weeks, months, and years went by as you grew to love the sailor in the wheelchair. He even told you on one occasion, that you were the "grandson he never had" and to, please, call him "Poppy." One fateful day, Poppy was trying to get out of bed and transfer himself to his wheelchair to go to the bathroom. However, his arms were still weak. Just as he was hoisting himself into the wheelchair, his arms collapsed, the wheelchair

ng, and so did Poppy. He landed face forward onto
You ran into his room, only to find him lying on the
; nose gushing bright red blood. He smiled apologeti-
cally with blood staining his teeth and trickling down his lips
and onto his shirt.

In that moment, love trumped your paralyzing fear of blood.
Instead of turning around and allowing the other nurses to deal
with it, like you usually did, you put on a pair of gloves, knelt
at Poppy's side, and placed a cold moist cloth over the bridge of
his nose to stop the flow of blood. You examined him in great
depth and miraculously found that a broken nose was the only
damage incurred. Poppy and you laughed and agreed that it was
his long history of hard work that had strengthened his bones,
and protected him from further damage that day.

Although it was actual bright red blood that dripped and
poured from Poppy's nose, your love for him blinded you from
being able to see the blood. You knew that you had a job to do,
and you did it. Just as mothers look past the blood coming from
their child's knees when they fall off of their bike in order to
nurture and care for them, you didn't see Poppy's blood that day.
You saw him hurting and had a deep desire to alleviate his pain.
Your love and compassion for him drove you to overcome your
fear of blood. You helped Poppy because that's what nurses do.

Deep red, flowing human blood is, in fact, the river of our
physical life. The fear of the sight of blood is a real phenomenon. However, there is another source of blood that is the river
of our eternal life. Jesus Christ! He overcame death, hell, and
the grave by His bloodshed. Before the death and Resurrection
of Jesus, the pure, undefiled blood of an animal had to be shed
in order to receive the forgiveness of our sins. However, Jesus
suffered a horrible death on a Cross between two criminals. His
physical blood flowed from His head, hands, feet, back, and
side. However, as His physical blood was visible and flowing,

unseen eternal blood was also flowing, as a sacrifice for our sins. Scripture reminds us that, "In him we have redemption through his [Jesus] blood, the forgiveness of our trespasses, according to the riches of his grace, which he lavished upon us, in all wisdom and insight, making known to us the mystery of his will, according to his purpose, which he set forth in Christ as a plan for the fullness of time, to unite all things in him, things in heaven and things on earth" (Ephesians 1:7–10).

So, when you think about pursuing nursing, remember it's all about the blood. Not literal blood, but eternal blood. Try not to allow the physical flow of blood to hinder you from fulfilling the calling that God may have placed on your life. Yes, you will encounter blood. At times, there may be extremely copious amounts of blood with which you are confronted. However, try to look beyond the physical "visual" blood, and look to the eternal "unseen" flow of blood. View your patients as vulnerable, hurting people that desperately need you. Serve them with a heart full of love and compassion, the same love and compassion that Christ demonstrated for us two thousand years ago on a Cross between two criminals.

My Prayer for You

Heavenly Father,

Thank You so much for the blood of Jesus Christ! Thank You for the sacrifice that You made so that we might have eternal life everlasting. Father, I pray for the person reading this book. If they have a fear of the sight of blood, I pray that You will put a filter over their eyes to only see the person behind the bleeding, and not the actual blood. Father, equip them with heavenly sight, to see the eternal blood that Jesus shed for them. Place a burden in their hearts for the sick and hurting. Show them how to help others and love like You do.

In Jesus' Holy and most precious name, Amen.

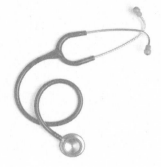

Chapter 4

A Legacy of Light

My father's words echoed through my mind as I recalled our recent phone conversation: "I have gone totally blind in my right eye! I can't even see any light. It is total darkness. This is really scary. Just close your eyes and imagine that darkness is all that you could see for the rest of your life." My dad had been receiving injections in his eyes to aid in decreasing the retinal edema that he had developed from years of uncontrolled diabetes and high blood pressure. Secondary to the injections, he had developed a staph infection in his right eye. The infection had caused him to go blind.

After hanging up the phone, I did as he instructed. I squinted both of my eyes tightly shut. Instant darkness. Absolute darkness. I could still smell the garlic and onions that my husband was cutting up in the kitchen in preparation for our dinner. I could hear the sound of my dog's feet scuffling across the hardwood floor and the buzz of the television in the background. I could feel the breeze from the ceiling fan blowing across my face and the softness of my bathrobe under my fingers. But I could not see anything. I could not even see so much as a hint of light. Sadness gripped my heart as I struggled to imagine a life without sight, a life without light. Luke 11:34 says: "Your eye is the lamp of your body. When your eye is healthy, your whole body is full of light, but when it is bad, your body is full of darkness." Again I closed my eyes and pondered darkness. I thought about never being able to gaze upon the beauty of the earth again, like seeing another magnificent golden sunset over the valley or a vibrant multi-colored rainbow after a thunderstorm. Tears welled up in my eyes as I tried to envision a life void of the ability to look into the faces of the people whom I love so deeply.

My mind began to drift off as I thought of the many people who were born into a world of blindness. They have never been blessed with the ability to physically see such beauty. They only get to imagine the sight of such wonders. Then I asked myself, what is vision? Is the gift of sight really physically seeing, or is it something deeper? What does it mean when the "whole body is full of light"?

Jesus Christ said, "I am the light of the world. Whoever follows me will not walk in darkness, but will have the light of life" (John 8:12). According to this passage, even a person born without sight can decide to follow Jesus, and no longer walk in darkness. Jesus becomes their light, and His light shines through them into the world. As nurses, we must not walk in darkness, but rather in the light of life, offering this light to our patients. "No one after lighting a lamp puts it in a cellar or under a basket, but on a stand, so that those who enter may see the light" (Luke 11:33). How true! The lamp in my living room is not there as a symbol of beauty to remain off at all times. No, it is there to be turned on as a source of light when the evening darkness approaches.

Florence Nightingale, one of the most influential figures in the nursing profession, lived out this Scripture to its fullest. She was often even referred to as the "lady with the lamp." Nightingale was born into an influential British family in the early 1800s. Much to her family's dismay, she turned down marriage proposals and a life of luxury in order to fulfill the calling that she believed God had placed on her life — the calling of becoming a nurse. In the 1850s, during the Crimean War, Nightingale weaved in and out of stretchers housing sick and dying soldiers in a hospital in Scutari, Turkey. Deep into the darkness of night, her lantern in hand, she would walk from soldier to soldier, offering herself as a loving, compassionate presence to those in need.

Nightingale observed with her eyes that these soldiers, known for their strength and valor, were stripped of their dignity, lying in their own urine and feces, without clean clothes, linens, water, or air. Cholera, typhoid fever, and the like were claiming their lives, rather than their wounds incurred from battle. As the soldiers lay in the physical darkness and filth, Nightingale observed with her heart that these soldiers were in desperate need of hope, in need of the light of life. Although Nightingale was a young nurse, she was a wise nurse. When she recognized a need, she worked diligently until that need was met.

Realizing the unsanitary conditions surrounding the soldiers were the root cause of many of their deaths, Nightingale led a team of nurses in improving the environment surrounding the soldiers. They scrubbed the wards from floor to ceiling. They opened the windows to allow in natural light and fresh air. Nightingale believed that fresh air and natural light were invaluable to the healing of the human body. In her book *Notes on Nursing*, she painted a picture of an uninhabited room where the air "has never been polluted by the breathing of human beings." She stated that in such a room, "you will observe a close, musty smell of corrupt air, of air i.e. unpurified by the effect of the sun's rays."[1] Furthermore, Nightingale and her team of nurses ensured that the soldiers' linens, clothes, and wound dressings were laundered regularly. When the sun set and the daylight turned to darkness, Nightingale would carry her lantern from soldier to soldier providing them with physical, emotional, and spiritual comfort. Because of Nightingale's valiant efforts, the hospital's death rate was reduced by two-thirds.

Today, if you walked into a hospital and witnessed conditions similar to Nightingale's observations in Turkey, what would you do? You would probably be appalled and report the facility to the authorities. Things such as clean air, fresh linens, and sterile wound dressings in United States hospitals are now an expectation, and are often taken for granted. Millions of dollars have been spent researching the effects of sanitation and environment on healing. We now have hundreds of various types of wound dressings and styles of dressing change procedures. However, healthcare and nursing are far from perfect.

Efforts must continually be made to ensure that patients receive the highest quality, latest evidence-based care. During the Crimean War, Nightingale challenged the status quo. She observed a need for something new, something different, and she ensured that it was completed. The light from her lamp became a symbol of hope and promise for the suffering soldiers. Nightingale emphasized that, "The most important practical lesson that can be given to nurses is to teach them what to observe — how to observe — what symptoms indicate improvement — what the reverse — which are of importance — which are of none — which are the evidence of neglect — and what kind of neglect."[2]

---

1. Florence Nightingale, *Notes on Nursing*, 1898, chapter 9, http://www.nursingplanet.com/nightingale/light.html.
2. Ibid., chapter 13.

Although Nightingale's ideals seem simplistic in today's nursing world, they are still very relevant. Technology is wonderful and necessary in healthcare. Lives are being saved secondary to revolutionary technological advances every day. However, the basic human need for light, love, and compassion remains. What we call "new" initiatives, such as the installation of windows in intensive care units (ICUs) to decrease psychosis among ICU patients, Nightingale demanded as necessary over 150 years ago. Patients should "be able, without raising themselves or turning in bed, to see out of window from their beds, to see sky and sun-light at least. . . ."[3] The profession of nursing must continue to reflect on Florence Nightingale's legacy of light. We must not be fearful to speak up when we see a need for change, no matter how simplistic or extravagant. We must show compassion for the human spirit, never hide our light under a basket, and place our lamp high on a lampstand for the entire world to see, so that nursing's legacy of light can live on into eternity.

My Challenge for You

Watch the video created by nurses and a multitude of professional nursing organizations entitled *If Florence Could See Us Now*. I believe that you will be touched and enlightened!

My Prayer for You

Heavenly Father,
You are the light of the world! Your eternal, heavenly light is the light of life. I pray that the person reading this book will have healthy eyes and a body full of light. Father, please allow Your light to shine through them. Give them the courage to place their lamp high on a lampstand for the entire world to see. I pray that when someone asks them from where their light and

---

3. Ibid., chapter 9.

joy comes, that they will not be fearful to share that it is from You. Father, I am grateful for the physical beauty of sunsets and rainbows, but more than that, I am thankful for the light that fills our bodies, Your light, the light of eternal life.

In Jesus' Holy and most precious name, Amen.

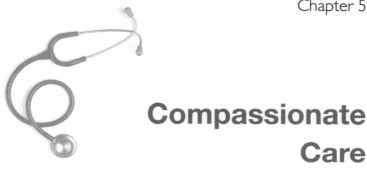

Chapter 5

Compassionate Care

Compassion is the sympathetic desire to alleviate another's discomfort and is motivated by deep, unconditional love. A nurse without compassion is like a car without a battery. It just does not work! Compassion is essential when caring for human beings in the most vulnerable states of life. Nursing void of compassion would simply be people checking things off of their "to do" list. Perhaps you or someone you love has encountered a nurse lacking compassion. If not, can you imagine a nurse without compassion?

Unfortunately, when I was a student nurse, I encountered an uncompassionate nurse. In fact, to this day, I have yet to encounter another one quite like her. I still get a lump in my throat and tears in my eyes when I think about the experience with this particular nurse. It was my junior year of my BSN program. Clinical rotations had just begun and I was exhilarated at the thought of taking care of patients in the hospital setting. A few of my classmates and I were assigned to a post-surgical floor in a relatively large hospital. We each only had one patient since we were just embarking on the hospital clinical nursing experience. My patient was an elderly woman who had recently undergone a radical abdominal surgery with colostomy placement. A colostomy is where a portion of the bowel is removed, and the intestine is pulled to the outside of the abdomen. The opening on the outside of the abdomen is called a stoma. The stoma allows feces to drain into a collection bag. It is actually a fairly routine procedure with a moderate recovery time, but this was not the case for my patient.

With my pen and clipboard in hand, I wrote furiously as I received the morning shift-to-shift nursing report. The night shift nurse informed me that, in addition to the recent surgery, my patient also had a history of diabetes and severe renal failure. Due to the severity of her renal failure, she was placed on dialysis to be completed several times per week. The nurse overtly expressed that, without dialysis, my patient would die. I swallowed hard the lump that had formed in my throat. The nurse's voice suddenly seemed far away as she continued explaining that my patient was extremely ill. She rattled off a list of specialists responsible for my patient's care, including a wound care specialist to manage her open abdominal wound. My heart pounded as I tried to focus on what she was saying. All I could think about was the extreme love and sympathy that I was feeling for the woman who was about to be entrusted to my care.

I snapped back to reality when the nurse began to explain how my patient's situation had gone from bad to worse. Following her surgery, the incision site on her abdomen had gotten infected. The infection brought massive amounts of swelling and inflammation around the incision site and throughout her body. This had caused the abdominal incision to dehisce and eviscerate. Dehiscence is when a wound does not heal properly and spontaneously opens. Evisceration is when internal organs protrude outside of the body through a dehiscence. In this case, my patient's incision was in the middle of her abdomen and spanned from just below her breastbone down to her navel. I winced as the nurse told me that since my patient's incision had dehisced and eviscerated, her intestines were completely exposed. Furthermore, she informed me that there was a clean dressing in place and that I should not touch it until the wound care nurse arrived.

When the nurse finally finished the report, I think I had to pick my jaw up off of the floor. She asked me if I had any questions. I thought to myself, "Oh my goodness! Questions! Yes, I have tons of questions. I have never seen a wound with intestines protruding out of a body before. I am just a student. What is it going to smell like? What should I say? What if I don't know what to do?!" However, all that I could muster myself to respond was, "No ma'am." And, with that, she turned around and walked away. Now, there I stood in my crisp hunter green uniform and pristine white lab coat with a million thoughts racing through my mind. My legs felt like gelatin as I pondered how to proceed. All morning, I prayed for the Lord to guide and direct my words, deeds, and actions throughout the day, and to please allow me provide compassionate, loving care to this woman, whatever that may look like.

After several minutes, I finally gathered up the strength and will power to walk into the patient's room. Instantly I was met with a smell that was unlike anything I had ever experienced. I continued putting one foot in front of the other until I could see around the corner. There she was, lying flat on her back staring at the ceiling. There were no visitors in her room. The sound of the TV buzzed in the background. As I got closer, I noticed how sad and lonely she appeared. I thought to myself, "This is someone's daughter. Someone's mother. Someone's sister. Someone's wife. She was created by God in His image." Instantaneously, all the fear and anticipation of being ill-equipped melted away. I finally reached her bedside, gently placed my hand over hers, and introduced myself as the student nurse who would be caring for her that day.

Throughout the morning, I strived to get to know my patient: who she was, where she was from, what her life was like before this hospitalization. She shared many of these things with me and more. We had countless sweet moments together as I assisted her with eating, bathing, and grooming. She shared with me her love for Jesus, how she hated her current situation, and that she just simply wanted to die. For the first time in my life, I was speechless. I had never encountered a patient who outwardly expressed their wish of dying before. This woman was allowing me into the most intimate details of her life. It was an honor and privilege, but I was scared. At barely 19 years old, and still a "baby nursing student," I pondered how I would ever be able to provide the care that this woman needed and deserved.

However, God had a plan, just as He always does. He was about to afford me the opportunity to provide the most compassionate care that I knew how to provide at that time. As the afternoon approached, the wound care nurse arrived on the unit to complete my patient's dressing change. I noticed right away that she was not going to be the "friendly type." Nonetheless, since I was eager to learn and glean all that I could from this process, I glued myself to her hip. When we entered the room I noticed my patient's demeanor instantly change. She was not the cheerful, willing woman with whom I had spent the morning. She had a look of paralyzing fear covering her face. I thought that it was probably due to the anticipation of the pain associated with the dressing change procedure. However, I was soon to find out that her fear was not only related to the pain and anguish caused by the procedure, but more so to do with the nurse performing it.

The wound care nurse militantly marched up to my patient's bed and, without so much as "hello," pulled back the sheets, raised up the patient's gown, and started the procedure. She was just checking things off of her "to do" list, completely void of compassion. I cringed as the nurse ripped off the tape and removed the old dressing with a huff. I am sure that my eyes were as big as saucers as I stared in disbelief at the gaping wound in the center of this sweet woman's abdomen. There were feces leaking in to the wound bed from the colostomy and it almost took my breath away. I tried to keep my composure and not allow my patient to see my uneasiness. The nurse hurriedly continued to scrub the wound, unfazed by the patient's groaning and crying. Her words were as sharp as a two-edged sword as she told my patient to "Hold still and quit whining. It can't hurt that bad!" There was no tenderness in the way that the nurse completed the procedure, or in the way that she spoke to my patient.

My heart ached as if it were my own family member lying in that bed! As I looked deeply into my patient's eyes, I not only saw pain and anguish, but I saw fear, undeniable fear. "Please, Lord, show me how to help this patient. Help me love her like You do. Help me provide her with compassionate care. Let her feel Your presence through me," I prayed. At that very moment, I did the only thing that I knew to do. I grabbed both of my patient's hands and held them in mine. I looked her straight in the eyes, and with tears streaming down my face, I began to softly sing "Amazing Grace." After the first few lines, she joined in with me. The wound care nurse continued to tug, pull, and huff and puff as my patient and I sang sweetly about the amazing grace of Jesus Christ.

Upon completion of the procedure, the wound care nurse gathered her things and exited the room, again with little to no acknowledgment of my patient. Following her exit, my patient smiled and thanked me for singing with her. She expressed how much it had helped ease her pain and occupy her mind during the dressing change. I told her it was my honor and privilege. Through the grace, power, and pure, undefiled love of Jesus Christ, I was able to overcome my own fears of inadequacy and inability, and demonstrate compassion to a lonely, scared woman at the mercy of those around her.

That afternoon, I told my nursing instructor about the unprofessional, unethical, and uncompassionate behavior of the wound care nurse. She further advocated on behalf of my patient, and reported it to the nursing supervisor. I do not know what happened to that nurse or whether she was disciplined or not. However, I do know that only hours after our encounter my patient decided to forego the continuation of dialysis. This meant that she was choosing to die. My initial reaction was to cry and throw my hands in the air and ask why. Then I realized, my patient's death would mean victory for her. She would no longer have to suffer or endure paralyzing pain and fear. She could rest. She would rest. She would be asleep in the Lord, and I would see her again.

But we do not want you to be uninformed, brothers, about those who are asleep, that you may not grieve as others do who have no hope. For since we believe that Jesus died and rose again, even so, through Jesus, God will bring with him those who have fallen asleep. For this we declare to you by a word from the Lord, that we who are alive, who are left until the coming of the Lord, will not precede those who have fallen asleep. For the Lord himself will descend from heaven with a cry of command, with the voice of an archangel, and with the sound of the trumpet of God. And the dead in Christ will rise first. Then we who are alive, who are left, will be caught up together with them in the clouds to meet the Lord in the air, and so we will always be with the

Lord. Therefore encourage one another with these words
(1 Thessalonians 4:13–18).

I pray that this story does not discourage you, but rather encourages you. I hope that you now see how compassion is mandatory in the profession of nursing. The patients entrusted to our care are in some of the most fragile and vulnerable states that they will ever experience. They allow us intimate views of their hearts if we will simply create a sacred place for them to do so. It is our obligation to provide patients with professional, ethically sound care. It is our honor and privilege, and should be our desire, to regard them as highly valuable and to tenderly and compassionately love them through it all.

My Prayer for You

Heavenly Father,

Thank You for being the perfect example of compassion. Thank You for my sweet patient who showed me that even the smallest deed can make a remarkable difference. Thank You for showing me what compassion does not look like, so that I can deepen my understanding of the compassion that You desire for me to have. I pray that the person reading this book intimately knows that You are the vine, and we are the branches, and without abiding in You we are unable to produce fruit, including compassion for our patients. Compassion cannot be taught. It must come from You. Father, give the reader of this book a deep understanding of true compassion and help them to daily realize Your love and compassion for them, so that they may offer that same unconditional, compassionate love to those entrusted in their care.

In Jesus' Holy and most precious name, Amen.

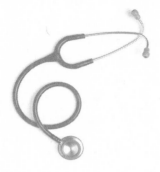

Sacrificial
Service

I sn't it refreshing to go into a restaurant in which the waiter or waitress goes above and beyond when waiting on your table? For instance, they speak with the head chef about preparing the food to meet your special dietary restrictions, they ensure that your glass of iced sweet tea never falls below the top of the rim, or they write a special "thank you" note on your receipt. I love it when my waiter or waitress smiles and engages in conversation with me. This demonstrates to me that they care about what they are doing — that what they are doing is more than just a job to them. The old adage "service with a smile" really does go a long way.

Many people base a waiter or waitress' tip on the quality of their service. What if nurses' salaries were based on the quality of our service? I wonder if the quality of our patient care would change. I can almost assure you that it would. If every nurse approached their patients with an attitude that sacrificial patient service was an honor and a privilege, I can guarantee you that the quality of patient care would skyrocket!

You can quit holding your breath now. Nursing salaries are not based on the quality of service which we provide. However, hospital reimbursement from the Center of Medicare and Medicaid Services is frequently based on customer satisfaction surveys. The Hospital Consumer Assessment of Healthcare Providers and Systems (HCAHPS) is a standardized national survey publicly presenting patients' perspectives of their hospital care. The majority of the survey scores are directly regarding the nursing care which the patients received. The survey allows patients to respond to questions regarding how well their nurses communicated with them, responsiveness to their needs, adequacy of their pain management, depth of communication regarding their medications, whether key information was provided at discharge, and whether or not they would recommend the facility to family and friends. Many hospitals post these results throughout their facility. Some unit managers actually post individual nurses names with their patient satisfaction scores for each category in table format on bulletin boards for all the other staff to view. Talk about motivation to provide quality care!

Please do not panic. I have been a nurse for over ten years, and have yet to receive a negative patient survey. This is certainly not because of my own human capabilities. All the glory belongs to God for His beautiful example of sacrificial service through Jesus Christ. Just as Jesus humbled Himself and scrubbed the filth from the feet of the disciples as an example to them, nurses must also treat their patients with the same kind of servant leadership. "As each has received a gift, use it to serve one another, as good stewards of God's varied grace" (1 Peter 4:10). Each time I walk into a patient's hospital room, nursing home suite, or their own home, I try to approach them as a child of God worthy of excellent service.

Excellent service in the nursing profession includes sacrificing: sometimes physical, sometimes emotional, sometimes

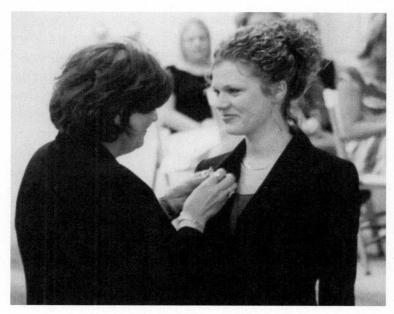

My mom pinning me at BSN Pinning Ceremony — "The
most important day of a nurse's life"

spiritual, and sometimes a combination of the three. But what
does it mean to sacrifice? To sacrifice means to give up, dedicate,
devote, yield, or surrender. You might be thinking that does not
sound so enticing or exciting. However, I can vouch that it is
enticing, exciting, and so much more. Nonetheless, you must be
in continuous communication with the Holy Spirit and willing
to relinquish all control to God.

Let's start with physical sacrifice. When I worked as a RN
on a medical-surgical floor, I was well acquainted with physical
sacrifice. I worked 12-hour night shifts from 6:30 p.m. until
7:00 a.m. Well, that was the supposed schedule. Many times
I would work into the 14th or 15th hour to ensure that all of
my patients were happy and settled, and that my charting was
completed with excellence. It was my preference to work five

consecutive shifts. This meant that I would work 60 or more hours without a night off. Some people thought I was crazy or that perhaps I had lost my mind. However, I loved for my patients to receive what we refer to as continuity of care. This meant that they would have the same nurse who knew their story, was aware of their condition, and could provide consistent care with regard to the patient, family, and provider's preferences for five nights in a row. By doing this, I could note whether or not my patients were improving or declining and devise a plan of care accordingly.

I cannot even begin to tell you how many pairs of white nursing shoes I destroyed from walking and standing for hours on end. At the end of each night I would check my pedometer. Seven miles or more was not unusual for the display to show. One night I remember looking at it and seeing 14 miles. That was a busy night! Physical sacrifice did not only consist of walking, standing, and wearing out shoes. There was also lifting and moving patients, as well as pushing and pulling heavy equipment, such as the crash cart. Oh, and don't forget about sleep. Sleep was a hot commodity! Working the night shift caused my circadian rhythm to become imbalanced, and when I did get a night off, it was difficult to sleep with the rest of world. I wanted to prowl all night and sleep all day.

Nonetheless, I adored working as a hospital medical-surgical nurse, especially working the night shift! If the Lord said that I had to go back to working on a hospital floor again tomorrow, I would choose the night shift all over again. It would take the remainder of this book to explain the rationale. So I will simply provide you with a few examples. There were countless times that I had the privilege of comforting a patient who was scared and could not find sleep. On many occasions, I prayed with families and friends who thought their loved one may die during the night.

Some of my patients had what is called "sundowners syndrome." This is where a person is lucid during the day, but at night they become very confused and may or may not become irritable and uncooperative. These were challenging patients, but challenges that I did not mind. It was so rewarding to be able to calm a confused patient and help them to find meaning and value. I distinctly remember one lady that was restless, could not sleep, and was completely confused. She had been spitting, cursing, and combative throughout the evening. Finally, we put her in a chair close to the nurse's station. I asked her if she would mind helping me with some laundry that I must get completed. She lit up like a Christmas tree. I brought several clean, unfolded towels and washcloths and placed them in front of her. That precious lady sat there for hours on end folding and refolding those towels and washcloths. She was neither upset nor combative for the remainder of my shift. She felt valuable and, deep inside, I felt good.

Physical sacrifice is something that nurses cannot avoid. Therefore, it is imperative that we find ways to replenish and rejuvenate ourselves. One way that I was able to continue the lengthy shifts night after night was to work five nights in a row and then have six nights off. It was like a mini-vacation every other week. This time allowed me to rest and refuel, not to mention sleep when the rest of the world slept. It also afforded me the opportunity to go out of town or spend time with my family and friends without ever having to request time off from my boss. Physical sacrifice can be taxing on the body. You must remember to take some time for yourself; time for rest and relaxation. This allows you to return to your patients, rejuvenated and ready to give of yourself once again, because they need you.

Physical sacrifice is not the only type of sacrifice that nurses endure when caring for patients. Emotional and spiritual sacrifice is also very evident and real within the profession of nursing.

We are continually offering ourselves as a compassionate presence to the sick and dying. On many occasions, I have sat with patients and families and cried. I believe they need to see this kind of emotion from their caregivers. This does not mean to cry uncontrollably with audible sobbing and snot running down your face. However, people need to know you care. You have probably heard the saying, "People don't care how much you know, until they know how much you care." This is very true!

It is a part of sacrificial service to allow our emotional side to reveal itself occasionally. It wasn't too long ago that I was checking on one of my nursing students in the neuro-trauma ICU. The charge nurse had assigned my student to a young male patient who had suffered an immense amount of brain swelling secondary to a motor vehicle accident. The patient was only 12 years old. The student informed me that she would be providing care for the patient and his family. Furthermore, she stated that the doctors had informed her that the child would never walk, talk, eat, or speak again, and that his new home would be a nursing care facility. Tears welled up in my eyes as I peered into his room. His body was lifeless with the exception of the machines breathing for him. My student and I took a moment to hug and cry apart from the family. I tried to encourage the student, but my heart was broken. The emotional sacrifice was getting the better of me. My student was actually stronger than I was in this situation. She said, "Don't worry Mrs. Harris, God is in control and He has got this!" My student went on that day and provided the most beautiful, intimate emotional and spiritual care for that patient and his family. I am sure that the Lord was smiling down that day and nodding in approval for my student's incredible sacrificial, emotional, and spiritual service.

You see, God gave us emotions. He even says to "weep with those who weep" (Romans 12:15), and that there is "a time to weep, and a time to laugh" (Ecclesiastes 3:4). I wept that day and have wept many more days throughout my career as a nurse. I am positive that I will weep an innumerable amount of times before my career has ended. However, I draw my strength from the Lord. I rely on Him to comfort me through the Holy Spirit when I am sad. When I am too weak to control the tears, and too devastated to find the words, He clears my mind and provides the words for me.

Physical, emotional, and spiritual sacrifice are inevitable in the nursing profession. However, the rewards are incredible! Something as simple as the words "thank you" from a patient is all that it takes to keep us going. And, on occasion, there are the most special of times when a wife of your patient finds you in Starbucks six years after you cared for her dying husband and tells you that "you were his angel disguised in a nurse's uniform." Those are the moments that all the sacrificial service you provide seems miniscule, but so worth it!

My Prayer for You

Heavenly Father,

Thank You so much for being the perfect example of sacrificial service. Thank You for being the well that doesn't run dry when we need physical, emotional, and spiritual replenishment. May Your example, Your love, and Your ultimate sacrifice on the Cross only deepen our desire to serve sacrificially those whom You have placed and will place in our nursing care. I pray that You will bless the reader of this book with a heart that yearns to serve others. May the people whom they serve see You working through them, using their hands, feet, mouths, and ideals to fulfill Your purpose.

In Jesus' Holy and most precious name, Amen.

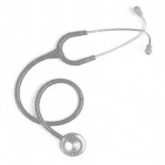

Chapter 7

Humble Heart, Helping Hands

ME, ME, ME! What about ME?! Sound familiar? Sadly, in today's society, we bake ourselves in tanning beds to get that golden bronze babe appearance, dye our hair to hide the gray, and bleach our teeth to decrease the coffee stains, all in order to enhance our outward beauty. We plaster *my kid is better than your kid* bumper stickers all over the rear end of our vehicles, and snap selfies with our smart phone cameras only to update our Facebook, Instagram, or Twitter statuses, as if the world cares. We live, work, and survive in a narcissistic, prideful, arrogant society. Although there is little room for these issues in our personal lives, there is even less room for pride and narcissism in the profession of nursing.

Life is fragile enough already. Combine that with the fact that healthcare is merely "practicing" interventions based on science and theory, and the fragility of life becomes overwhelmingly increasingly evident. Nonetheless, on various occasions throughout my career, I have encountered healthcare professionals who were convinced that they were on a level playing field with God. On rare occasions, I have actually witnessed one or two of them verbalizing this very thing to patients. It is not only appalling, but dangerous territory in which to be treading. Proverbs 16:18 says, "Pride goes before destruction, and a haughty spirit before a fall."

I am convinced that if we were to delve deeper into the root issue behind most medication errors, wrong-site surgeries, and patient/resident negligence injuries, we would find that prideful, haughty spirits played a vital role. You cannot even turn on the television anymore without some lawyer advertising their services to defend individuals against healthcare-related injuries. If we, as healthcare professionals, followed the example of Christ and did nothing from rivalry or conceit, but in humility counted others more significant than ourselves (Philippians 2:3), there would be no need for such legal representation.

Jesus Christ was the King of kings and the Lord of lords. He could have sat on a throne high above the rest of the world, adorned with a crown of gold and a robe of royalty. Yet He counted the entirety of mankind as more significant than Himself. He did not even have to associate with the lowly, but He chose to surround Himself with them. He exercised undeniable humility as He was publicly persecuted, cursed, spat at, beaten beyond recognition, and ultimately murdered as a sacrifice to offer redemption for mankind. Nurses could learn a few things from Jesus' example.

Too often, we get caught up in promotions, titles, and earning the alphabet behind our name. We think that licenses and certifications somehow elevate us above others; or, perhaps, the pins dangling from our name badges are indicative of the possession of superhero powers. Although education is a powerful tool, and certifications strengthen our professional practice, we must not allow ourselves to become so haughty or prideful that we lose sight of the calling that God has placed upon our lives: to love and serve others. Continually asking God to preserve our humility and to keep us grounded in truth is necessary. Reminding ourselves that we are simply vessels of the Holy Spirit being used as instruments to fulfill the will of God has to be a daily practice. It is our human nature to seek the approval of others. We want to know that we are doing well and that other people are impressed with our accomplishments and work.

Jesus says to "encourage one another and build one another up" (1 Thessalonians 5:11). However, when the approval of others supersedes the approval of God in our eyes, building one another up becomes a sport of *fishing for compliments* to feed our own arrogance. Thus, we risk crossing the line between confidence and cockiness. This type of behavior can permeate an organization faster than the smell of burnt microwave popcorn.

You have probably heard the saying that "one bad apple can spoil the whole bunch." Well, the same concept applies to nursing. It only takes one nurse with an arrogant, holier-than-thou attitude to shift the morale of an entire unit, especially if that nurse is in a leadership position. However, the same is true of a nurse leader exemplifying kind, humble characteristics.

There is a small nursing home situated on a beautiful riverbank in southern Missouri. I have to tell you that this is not just any nursing home. It happens to be the most incredible nursing home I have ever had the privilege of visiting. I first entered this facility five years ago as the clinical instructor for a group of junior nursing students. Within moments of stepping across the threshold of the massive magnificent wooden front door, I recognized that something was different.

The first person that I encountered was the receptionist. She greeted me with a genuine smile and warmly welcomed me to their facility. As I peered down the hallway, I noticed paintings and pictures lining the walls. It felt warm and cozy. When my eyes cast downward to the floor, they were so clean that I bet you could have eaten off of them. As I advanced down the hallway, I recognized a smell unfamiliar to nursing homes. It was that of fresh fragrant flowers and bleach. It smelled clean! I was shocked that there was not even a hint of the typical nursing home smells, such as the strong ammonia odor from the infrequent changing of the residents' incontinence briefs.

I followed the pleasant smell around the corner. A short, jolly, gray-haired lady glanced up from mopping. As soon as we made eye contact, she, like the receptionist, smiled genuinely and spoke to me like we were long lost friends. It was almost as if I could feel the joy radiating from her body. It was obvious that she did her job as if unto the Lord. I later learned that the sweet jolly lady was 76 years old and, instead of retiring, chose to continue working in the facility because of her love for the administrators, staff, and residents. Wow! You don't hear that about a nursing home very often, or about any organization for that matter.

Momentarily, I thought I might be hallucinating. This is because almost every nursing home in which I have ever worked or visited did not have the warm, welcoming, homey atmosphere that this one had. More often, they had cold concrete cinder-block walls, stale unpleasant air like that of a dirty diaper, and if I could ever locate a staff member, their standoffish dispositions and unwillingness to help was like staring into the eyes of a tree full of hoot owls. Not this facility!

Five years have gone by since I first entered the nursing home on the river. The staff, from the administrators to the environmental service professionals, still treats the residents like their own family. There is consistently a waiting list for those trying to become residents. Through my time in the facility, I believe that I have discovered the recipe behind such a successful operation. Humility!

First of all, the owners/administrators are present every day. They genuinely and lovingly interact with the staff and residents. Only on rare occasion are they even in their offices. The dining hall and residents' rooms are where they spend the majority of their time throughout the workday. Successful leaders lead by example. I distinctly remember one occasion when I was working with a nursing student. We were gathering supplies to provide care to a resident when we happened to pass a facility administrator. This particular administrator also carries the titles of registered nurse and follower of Jesus Christ. I turned my head to examine what the student was staring at in disbelief. A smile came across my face as I observed the most beautiful sight. My body felt warm and fuzzy inside as I watched that administrator humbling herself. In her freshly laundered, crisp dress clothes, she was joyfully mopping up the urine of a resident that had experienced a moment of incontinence.

She could have asked a nurse, a nursing assistant, or an environmental service professional to complete the job that many would consider menial. However, she chose to lead by example and do it herself. My student was astonished. I was thrilled! The humility demonstrated by this administrator trickled down into every individual working throughout the facility. I once observed the maintenance man searching for chocolate ice cream for a resident who did not want the vanilla which was stocked at that time. It was heartwarming and precious to see the amount of effort this gentleman put forward to ensure the resident received her request. The maintenance man was not too good to honor the needs of others. He had seen humility modeled by the leaders of the facility and embodied that same humility to serve the residents in any way that he found necessary.

I could go on forever about every staff member in the nursing home on the river. The majority of the employees have worked there an average of 7 years. I personally know of three nursing assistants who have been there 20 or more years! That speaks volumes about the work environment created by the leaders, especially when there is a 70 to 100 percent turnover rate among nursing assistants working in nursing care facilities across the United States.[1]

This is only one example supporting humility as an important aspect of nursing, but I believe a powerful one. In a society driven by success, fortune, and fame, it is difficult to remain humble. Humility is a choice! I pray that on your journey to nursing, you will recognize the sanctity and sacredness of the profession, and that you will continuously regard others as more valuable than yourself. This does not mean that you must surrender the characteristics that comprise the breadth and depth of who you are. However, it does afford you the opportunity to find joy in your work as you bless others.

My Prayer for You

Heavenly Father,

Thank You for people who choose to lead with humility. Thank You for showing me what humble leadership looks like. You were the most beautiful example of humility as You gave up Your life to save mine. What an unselfish, humble act of love. Please help me to remain humble and count others as more valuable than myself as I continue this important calling of nursing. I pray that the reader of this book will also exercise humility as they continue their journey to nursing. If they discover that nursing is not the profession to which You are calling them, I ask that You aid them in continued humility as they work toward another profession.

In Jesus' Holy and most precious name, Amen.

---

1. A. Hussain and P.A. Rivers, "Confronting the Challenges of Long-term Health Care Crisis in the United States," *Journal of Healthcare Finance* (2009), 36, 71–82, retrieved from http://web.ebscohost.com/ehost/pdfviewer/pdfviewer?vid=17&sid=b76b8f38-6d02-45a8-9d4f-41528136 7ad8%40sessionmgr115&hid=108.

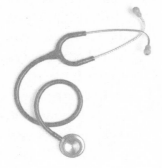

Chapter 8

Integrity Is Integral

When thinking about the most important characteristics that a nurse must possess, one cannot forget to include integrity. C.S. Lewis is quoted as saying, "Integrity is doing the right thing, even when no one is watching."[1] Have you ever done something that was dishonest, unethical, or illegal, simply because you could? Or maybe you have known someone who has. Unfortunately, my heart was recently broken due to someone's lack of integrity. This person is someone I love very much and who actually loves me too. However, entitlement and personal desire superseded their self-control in the moment. When no one was watching, this person set integrity aside and decided to steal from me.

Even the kindest, most loving, and typically honest person can be riddled with confusion and jeopardize their integrity in a moment of desperation. As I read the Missouri State Board of Nursing report each quarter, I am reminded of this very thing. At the end of the board report, there is page after page of nursing

---

1. http://www.brainyquote.com/quotes/quotes/c/cslewis700208.html.

disciplinary actions and licensure probations and revocations that happened during the previous few months. It deeply saddens me as I read the stories of nurses diverting drugs from the facilities in which they are employed, abusing residents in nursing care facilities, or consistently making critical errors and not reporting them appropriately. These are only a few examples. Sadly, there are numerous more. No matter the offense, there is one commonality spiraled throughout each of these stories. They all include nurses — human beings who chose to abort morals, values, ethics, and integrity, and when no one was watching, did the wrong thing.

This is not a new phenomenon. Humans have struggled with integrity from the beginning of time. Adam and Eve were deceived and driven by curiosity and selfish desire in the Garden of Eden. In a moment's time, through one action, mankind fell and sin entered the world. Thus, we must consistently be on high alert, maintaining self-control, so as not to be deceived.

Nurses are some of the most trusted and valued professionals on earth. From the moment a nurse walks into a patient's room, there is a level of trust that exists. Patients and their families commission nurses as sound decision-makers and individuals with exceptional morals, values, and ethical standards. What patients and families tend to forget is that nurses are not supernatural. We do not possess superhuman powers or strengths. Just like Adam and Eve, we face the same challenges and temptations as the remainder of the world.

Think about what you would do in the following situation. You are strolling down the sidewalk on a sunny autumn morning. The temperature is in the mid-70s. The sun is beaming down on your face with the perfect amount of intensity. Soft, melodic musical tones from Norah Jones' latest album are streaming through your earbuds. Your mind cannot help but reflect on your plans for the future. It has always been your dream to travel across the country and stay in every bed and breakfast along the way, but you do not even own a car. With transportation, housing, and food expenses, you could not possibly ever see this dream come to fruition. All of a sudden your thoughts come to a screeching halt as you lose your balance and nearly fall face first into the pavement. What in the world did you trip over? You look down. There, lying on the sidewalk glistening in the sun, is the solution to all of your problems. It is a shiny black wallet just lying there, waiting for someone to pick it up and claim it as their own. Inside you find over $3000.00 in cash, and one of each of the major credit cards. You think to yourself, there is probably at least $10,000.00 worth of credit on each card. You ponder all of the things that you could do with this much cash and credit!

Okay, let's get back to reality. Although this is an improbable scenario, you are at an ethical crossroad. What would you do in this situation? Would you take the cash and throw the wallet into the bushes and act like nothing ever happened? Take the cash and the credit cards and go on a major online shopping spree? Keep the cash and turn the wallet with the remaining items into the local police station? Or would you look through the wallet to see if there was a driver's license and an address to return the wallet and all of its contents to the rightful owner? So many choices, but which choice includes integrity?

The obvious honest choice is to look through the wallet and try to return it with the cash and all other contents intact to the rightful owner. This may seem like a far-fetched scenario, but let's think about a similar scenario related to the nursing profession. Now, you are a nurse working the night shift in a busy nursing care facility. No one is aware, but your mother is suffering from intractable pain related to severe bone cancer. She lives with you, does not have insurance, and cannot afford her pain medication. You know that she is dying and you desperately want her last few weeks on earth to be peaceful, but without pain medication, peace is not an option. At work, you are in charge of all medication administration, including narcotics. You know that the narcotics are locked in the medication room and you are one of the nurses with a key. Every narcotic medication has to be counted and manually signed out each time one is administered. When a nurse removes a capsule or tablet, the amount removed and the amount remaining must be documented.

Today, as you are preparing to administer one of the resident's oxycodone tablets, you notice that there is a discrepancy in the previous documentation. It says that there should be seven tablets remaining, but there are really ten. It is like those extra three tablets do not even exist. No one will ever know if you take them home and give them to your mom to help ease some of her pain during her final moments on earth. You think to yourself that it would be an act of mercy.

Okay, freeze! Although there is a discrepancy and it might not ever be discovered that you take those three oxycodone tablets, it is still dishonest and considered theft. Integrity does not only include honesty, it also includes justice and doing what is right even when others may say it is wrong. For instance, if you noticed a baby sleeping, strapped into a car seat in a boiling hot car with all of the windows up and there was absolutely no one around to help you, what would you do? Would you turn your head and walk on by since it would be considered destruction of property if you broke a window and got the baby out of the car; or would you smash the window out with whatever tool that you could get your hands on and rescue the child? A person of great integrity would not worry about the consequences of breaking the car window. They would do what is right — rescue the baby.

Let's think about another nursing-related scenario. What if you were working on the evening shift at a small hospital and you notice that one of your colleagues reeks of alcohol. When you confront the person, they state that they are sober and only had a couple of drinks prior to their shift. You know that, if they are sent home, you will have to take care of your patients and theirs until a replacement nurse arrives. Although your colleague's speech is slightly slurred, you know that they are not drunk, and are confident that they could still do their job with little difficulty. Nonetheless, you know that it is against hospital policy to be under the influence of any amount of alcohol when on the clock. What do you do? A person with integrity would not be concerned with the relationship strain that may arise between themselves and their colleague. They would follow the facility policy and report the person in order to protect the safety of the patients entrusted to their care.

Let's examine one more scenario. You are a registered nurse working in an outpatient clinic. All the other staff, with the exception of the physicians and the office manager, report directly to you. As you walk past the nurses' station, you overhear several medical assistants giggling and bantering about how they performed a drug screen on one of your patients without the patient's consent. They are whispering loudly enough that you hear them discussing the large number of illegal substances that were present in the patient's specimen. When confronted, the medical assistants admit to completing the drug screen without the patient's consent. They explain that they knew the patient was addicted to illegal drugs and that they performed the test simply because they were bored and wanted some entertainment.

You have a choice, you could verbally reprimand the medical assistants, throw away the test results, and act like nothing ever happened, or you could verbally explain the severity of the actions and potential consequences to the medical assistants, as well as complete an incident report to be submitted to the administrators of the clinic. Then the punishment for the incident would be determined by your supervisors. Obviously, the right choice is option number two. You were the licensed professional in charge and you must maintain the integrity of your profession and the clinic. If the patient was made of aware of the incident and discovered that the clinic policy was not followed, legal ramifications could ensue.

These are only a handful of examples that include dilemmas requiring honesty and integrity. If you choose to enter into the profession of nursing, I am positive that you will encounter innumerable more. You have a choice: to be a person of integrity or not. Your choices can affect your licensure, your livelihood, and the lives of others. God desires us to be men and women of honesty and integrity. Throughout the years, I have been able to maintain my integrity by reminding myself that, when no one else is watching, God is watching. I try to envision Jesus standing beside me, peering over my shoulder. Then, when I make an error, choosing not to report it does not even seem like an option. So I pray that when you are faced with adversity and the easy way out looks so enticing, you will ask yourself what you would do if Jesus was standing before you in the flesh.

My Prayer for You

Heavenly Father,

You are a God of mercy and love, but also a God who desires honesty and integrity. You are our Father and You desire each of Your children to honor You in every aspect of our lives. This includes our minds, hearts, and actions. Please help me to be a woman of integrity, always choosing to do the right thing, even when no one is watching. Father, I pray that the reader of this book will also be a person of great integrity. Each

time they face an ethical crossroad, whether in the nursing profession or elsewhere, I pray that they will always
choose the high road — the road to integrity. Lord,
help us all to make godly, wise decisions that will maintain not only our own integrity, but the integrity of the
Kingdom of God.

In Jesus' Holy and most precious name, Amen.

Chapter 9

Communication and Collaboration: Critical Care

People often use the words "communication" and "collaboration" synonymously. However, they are not synonyms. To communicate simply means using words, sounds, signs, or behaviors in order to get your point across; whereas to collaborate means to work with another person or a team to achieve a goal.[1] Even tiny babies communicate by crying when they are hungry, sleepy, have a dirty diaper, or are experiencing pain. It is difficult to determine what a baby needs simply by their cry. Thus, you must monitor their body language to determine the reason behind the cry. For instance, arching the back and stiffening the body usually indicates that they are experiencing flatulence or gas; or if they are just whimpering and rubbing their eyes, they need to be put to bed because they are sleepy.

Communication among adults is not much different. Ninety-three percent of adult communication is non-verbal, including body language and tone of voice. This leaves only

---

1. Merriam- Webster Online Dictionary, http://www.merriam-webster.com/.

seven percent of all communication for actual words or sounds.[2] In other words, it really does not matter *what* a person says, but, more so, *how* they say it. So my husband will be more apt to take out the trash if I politely request that he do so while smiling, holding a relaxed posture, and keeping my tone of voice calm and even, rather than asking him to take the trash out in a sarcastic tone of voice with my hands on my hips while rolling my eyes. This concept plays a critical role in the profession of nursing, as well as healthcare in general. The manner in which a person communicates also affects the success of their collaboration with patients, families, and other members of the healthcare team.

If the majority of communication is non-verbal, then the manner in which you approach others, especially during a first encounter, can make or break a relationship. I am a huge advocate for making a good first impression. Think about a job interview. Would you rather hire the person who saunters arrogantly into your office with their hair and clothes disheveled, plops down into a chair, is unable to make eye contact, answers questions aloofly while popping their gum and fidgeting with their phone; or would you rather hire the person that walks into your office in a crisp laundered suit, firmly shakes your hand and introduces themselves, sits when asked, keeps their body language open without crossing their arms, and answers your questions with confidence while maintaining eye contact? Even if both of these individuals received the same interview questions and answered with exactly the same words, I feel sure that most people would be more apt to hire the latter, rather than the former. This is because non-verbal communication is critical.

Imagine that you are a 26-year-old female patient named Ruth. You are lying in a hospital bed, desperate for answers. The doctor recently broke the news to you and your family that

---

2. James Borg, *Body Language: How to Know What's Really Being Said*, (Harlow, England: Pearson, 2012).

you are dying of cancer. It all finally sank in yesterday and you sobbed most of the evening. Today, you have experienced horrific nausea and vomiting from the high-dose chemotherapy. It has been so intense that your head is pounding, your mouth feels like the Sahara desert, your palms are clammy, your heart is racing, and really, you just feel miserable. Think about the nurse you would rather have caring for you that evening. Nurse #1 walks up to your bed, places a hand lightly over yours, softly introduces herself (or himself) with an empathetic facial expression, and asks what she can do to alleviate your discomfort. Nurse #2 barges into your room still laughing loudly, secondary to the conversation that she just completed in the hallway, hands you an emesis basin with a look of disgust on her face, crosses her arms over her chest, and as she is backing toward the exit, asks what she can do for you. Although both nurses offered the same assistance, it is probably a no-brainer that you would choose nurse #1. Nurse #1's body language implied that she cared about you and that she was willing to collaborate with you on your treatment plan, whereas nurse #2's body language demonstrated hurriedness and a lack of concern.

Let's pretend that compassionate nurse #1 is the nurse assigned to you and that her name is Kristin. Kristin obviously has therapeutic communication skills, but what about the ability to collaborate? Let's go back to your hospital room. Later in the evening, a million thoughts are racing through your mind as you contemplate your life and what to do next. Your heart is breaking thinking about what is going to happen to you. How long do you have left to live? Should you have the surgery to try to remove the tumor on your brain? Will you lose control of your bodily functions? Will you forget your family? Will dying be painful? How will you pay for all of the medical expenses? Where will your spirit go after you die? It feels like a melting pot of emotions.

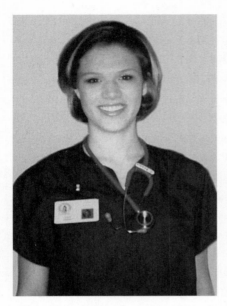

First clinical day of nursing school at Arkansas Tech University

Kristin walks into the room with her calm yet warm demeanor. She can sense that you are upset. She pulls up a chair next to your bed and simply listens as you shower your concerns down on her like a rainstorm. When you pause for a moment due to the tears cutting off your ability to speak, Kristin reaches over and pulls a tissue from the box. She gently places the tissue in your hand and gives you a reassuring glance. As you are wiping the tears from your face and blowing your nose, Kristin assures you that she is there to be your advocate and to collaborate with each and every member of the healthcare team so that you receive the highest quality of care. You know in your heart that she is speaking the truth, but suddenly her voice becomes muffled. The room begins spinning around you. The lights grow distant and dim. You can hear Kristin shouting your name, but you are unable to answer. In an instant everything goes black.

Kristin leaps into action. She begins checking your pulse and respirations, and communicating with the nursing assistant. She instructs the nursing assistant to collect your vital signs while she completes a quick physical exam. You can feel the cold stethoscope moving from place to place over your chest. You sense the blood pressure cuff inflating and squeezing your left arm, but you are still unable to move. You hear

Kristin communicating with the nursing assistant that your vital signs are stable right now, but that your heart is beating rapidly and your blood pressure is beginning to decline. Suddenly, you feel the bed changing positions. Your head is now pointed toward the floor and your feet are in the air. Kristin explains to the nursing assistant that she has placed you in trendelenberg position to assist the blood flow to your brain. The two healthcare professionals collaborate in hushed tones for a few more seconds, and then Kristin leaves the room. The nursing assistant remains at your bedside checking vitals for what seems like every five seconds.

At the nurses' station, Kristin quickly glances back over your labs. She notices that your electrolytes are imbalanced. She knows that if they get any worse there could be severe consequences. She also knows that approximately 60 percent of critical medical errors are related to telephone miscommunication.[3] Therefore, Kristin allows the words and emotions from your conversation and the current events to replay over and over in her mind, prior to contacting your physician. The best way to collaborate urgent or emergent matters within the healthcare team is to keep it simple. Just as Jesus communicated in simplistic, short stories called parables, healthcare team members follow a similar, simplistic methodology through a standardized form of communication called SBAR(R). SBAR(R) allows individuals to present information in an unbiased manner, and encourages collaboration. In a matter of a single minute, Kristin jots some notes onto the SBAR(R) form before she makes the call. SBAR(R) stands for Situation, Background, Assessment, Recommendation, and Response. Not only does SBAR(R) enhance and streamline communication and collaboration, it also decreases the anxiety

3. H.P. Katz, D. Kaltsounis, L. Halloran, and M. Mondor, "Patient Safety and Telephone Medicine," 2008, http://www.ncbi.nlm.nih.gov/pmc/articles/PMC2324141/.

associated with calling physicians, and, most importantly, promotes patient safety.

Kristin struggles to keep her hand from trembling as she dials the four-digit extension. She places the phone receiver to her ear and waits for the ringing to subside. After the third ring, the on-call physician answers. Kristin begins the conversation by explaining the *Situation*: "Good evening. My name is Kristin and I am the nurse taking care of Ruth in room number 140. I am calling because approximately five minutes ago, Ruth passed out while I was sitting at her bedside." Then, Kristin briefly explains the *Background*: "Ruth is a 26-year-old female recently diagnosed with a malignant brain tumor. She has been receiving high-dose chemotherapy and was admitted to the hospital four days ago for weakness, dizziness, and blurred vision. She has been vomiting off and on all evening. Her vital signs have been stable throughout my shift; however, following this episode her pulse increased to 115 beats per minute and her blood pressure decreased to 98/62. That is a significant change from her baseline. Her potassium is high at 5.8 and her sodium is low at 125. I placed her in trendelenberg position and the nursing assistant is in the room with her, obtaining vital signs every five minutes." Kristin further explains her *Assessment* of the current situation: "I believe that Ruth is dehydrated from all of the nausea and vomiting." The physician acknowledges Kristin's concerns with compassion in her tone.

Kristin then states her *Recommendation*: "I really believe that Ruth needs some fluid replacement via intravenous (IV) infusion." The physician *Responds* in agreement with Kristin's assessment and recommendations, compliments her on the quick, thorough assessment and communication, orders IV fluids and nausea medication to be started immediately, and encourages Kristin to call back if Ruth is not improving over the next 30 minutes.

Following the administration of IV fluids and nausea medication, you are feeling much better. Secondary to efficient, effective communication and collaboration between the nurse, nursing assistant, and physician, your head is no longer pounding, the room is quiet and still, and you can see, hear, and communicate without difficulty. Your heart is grateful that Kristin was able to communicate and collaborate with other valuable healthcare team members in order to best care for you. You know that this is just the beginning of a long journey full of medications, hospitals, and nurses. However, thanks to Kristin, you feel confident that all of your future physical, emotional, and spiritual needs will be met. When everyone has left the room, you close your eyes and silently thank God for the simplistic way in which He communicated with His disciples, and Kristin's ability to follow that example.

My Prayer for You

Heavenly Father,

Thank You for words, sounds, and the ability to speak. Thank You for knowing that humans desperately need communication and human interaction, both verbal and non-verbal. It seems logical that the majority of our communication is non-verbal. As humans, we often speak the words "I love you," but our non-verbal communication says otherwise. Father, I ask that You bless both the reader and me with the ability to communicate effectively and collaborate as team members in the Body of Christ so that we may communicate love more effectively. Although nurses are often the individuals spending the most time with patients and are central to patient care, without the healthcare team, and effective communication and collaboration, patient conditions would rapidly deteriorate. You say in Your

Word, "For just as the body is one and has many members, and all the members of the body, though many, are one body, so it is with Christ" (1 Corinthians 12:12). Father, I ask You to remind us often that teamwork makes the dream work.

In Jesus' Holy and most precious name, Amen.

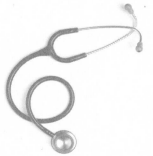

Chapter 10

Organization Is
Not Optional

Baking a cake seems like a pretty simplistic endeavor, at least when using a boxed cake mix. However, if you do not gather your supplies before you begin, you may get to the part where you whisk in the eggs, only to discover that you are completely out of eggs. Well, you know as well as I do that without eggs there is no cake! Just like eggs are not optional when making a cake, organization is not optional when caring for patients.

At 6:00 a.m., 30 minutes prior to the start of her shift, Vickie walked into the medical unit at the local community hospital where she had recently started her new job as a registered nurse. As always, she was eager and excited to see what adventure the day would hold. As she hung her purse and jacket on the hook in her locker, she closed her eyes and asked the Holy Spirit to give her direction throughout the long 12-hour shift ahead of her. She picked up her clipboard, placed a few papers under the clip, shut her locker, and secured the combination lock in place. She smiled as she ran her fingers across the pictures of her husband and children covering the front of the blue-metal door. They were her entire world. She kept pictures of them on her locker to remind her to be the kind of nurse she desired for them to have if the day ever arrived when they should need one.

At 6:10 a.m., Vickie sat down, scooted her chair under the break room table, and pulled a multi-colored ink pen from her scrub shirt pocket. She glanced over her nursing report papers. She had created a report sheet template when she was in nursing school and had used it ever since. The report sheet was on standard 8.5" x 11" printer paper and was divided into six sections. Six sections worked well, except on occasion when she had seven patients. In those instances, she used two report sheets. In each section of the paper, there was a place for the patient's room number, name, primary and secondary diagnoses, diet, mobility, IV site and type of fluid, abnormal lab values, vital signs, and a comment section to jot down any significant changes noted by the nurse on the previous shift. Vickie folded the report sheet over the clipboard and checked to make sure that the most current insulin and heparin protocols were easily accessible, since many of her patients were on these particular medications.

At 6:15 a.m., the unit charge nurse walked into the break room and assigned Vickie her patients. Today she would only have five patients, since a few of them were very acute and others needed some extra TLC. Vickie carefully wrote down each patient's name, diagnosis, and doctor on her report sheet in black ink. Patient #1 was Mr. Louis, a 96-year-old male WWII veteran admitted for an exacerbation of heart failure. Patient #2 was a 19-year-old female with staph infection secondary to a spider bite on her forearm. Vickie noted that she requested to be called by her first name, Sarah. Nurses should always refer to their patients by Mr. or Ms. and the patient's last name, until the patient requests otherwise. This is a form of respect. Vickie wrote the name Sarah in the appropriate box and circled it in blue ink to remind her of this request. Vickie's third patient was Mr. Smith, a 46-year-old homeless male that slept under bridges and on local park benches prior to this hospital admission. Three days ago, he was found drunk and passed out in front of a shopping mall and brought to the hospital by emergency medical personnel. Patient #4 was Mrs. Carol, a 60-year-old female admitted with intractable back pain secondary to a recent work-related injury. The fifth and final patient assigned to Vickie was a 72-year-old male patient named Mr. Hill. Mr. Hill was admitted for anemia from a severe lower gastrointestinal bleed.

After Vickie wrote down this basic information, she quickly walked to the nurse's station, logged into an available computer, and pulled up each of her patient's electronic health records. Since shift report would not begin until 6:30 a.m., she had 15 minutes to review the morning lab results and note any significant changes in the overnight vital signs. Vickie noticed Mr. Hill's anemia had worsened over the last two days. His hemoglobin had dropped significantly, and Vickie was sure that he would need a blood transfusion on her shift. The only other significant lab value that Vickie noted was Sarah's white blood cell count. It was declining, indicating that she was positively responding to the antibiotic therapy. Vickie wrote down each of the abnormal lab values in red ink to indicate significant information pertinent to the care which she would provide to her patients.

At 6:30 a.m., Vickie met the nurse responsible for each of her patients on the previous shift. The nursing shift-to-shift report ended at 7:05 a.m. Vickie glanced down at her clipboard and her notes, and took one last quick glance at the electronic health records to verify any medications or procedures that required urgent completion. Vickie organized her thoughts and prioritized which patient would need care first, second, third, and so on. She determined that Mr. Hill would need to be seen first since his blood levels had dropped overnight, indicating that his gastrointestinal bleed was worsening. Vickie also noted that Sarah's antibiotic would need to be administered promptly at 8:00 a.m. to ensure that the medication remained at a therapeutic level in her bloodstream. Vickie wrote a large "#1" next to Mr. Hill's name and made a note regarding the antibiotic in bright red in Sarah's section on her report sheet.

Vickie visited Mr. Hill and noted that he was alert and oriented to person, place, time, and situation. He was following the physician's dietary orders of "nothing by mouth" religiously so that he could have his colonoscopy completed that morning. Vickie had Mr. Hill sign the surgical consent form. She collaborated with the nursing assistant regarding the completion of Mr. Hill's tap water enemas until they were clear and made her nursing notes in the computer at the bedside. It was officially 7:20 a.m. when Vickie entered Mrs. Carol's room to check her morning blood sugar and administer her IV pain medication. Since Mrs. Carol's blood sugar was within the normal range, she did not require any insulin at that time. Vickie noted this in the electronic medication administration record and at 7:45 a.m. went on to the next patient.

Mr. Louis was sitting up in bed eating his breakfast when Vickie walked into the room. Vickie quickly assessed his mental, respiratory, and cardiovascular status. She called the telemetry technician to get a report as to what the heart monitor was reading. Mr. Louis was in a normal sinus rhythm with an occasional irregular beat called a premature ventricular contraction. Vickie knew that she would need to keep a close eye on Mr. Louis' fluid intake and output, so she jotted down how much fluid he had drunk with his breakfast in green ink on her report sheet. Just as Vickie was about to exit the room, Mr. Louis voiced that he needed to go to the bathroom. Remembering the difficulty that the previous nurse iterated about Mr. Louis' ability to ambulate, she turned around and assisted Mr. Louis to the bedside commode.

By this time it was getting close to 8:00 a.m. and Sarah would need to have her antibiotics hung and infusing very soon. Thus, Vickie handed Mr. Louis his call light and instructed him to press the red button when he was finished using the bedside commode. She further educated him not to attempt getting up without assistance as a protective mechanism against falls. In order to best utilize time and resources, Vickie delegated that the nursing assistant be on alert for Mr. Louis' call light and to assist him as quickly as possible when he was ready to go back to bed. Furthermore, Vickie reminded the nursing assistant to document the amount of urine in Mr. Louis' measuring device prior to leaving the room. The nursing assistant gladly accepted the delegation because she knew that she was a valuable member of the healthcare team, and that Vickie had to complete more complex duties that were outside of a nursing assistant's scope of practice.

Vickie entered the medication room with a swipe of her badge and located the antibiotic that was to be infused to fight Sarah's staph infection. Vickie also made a mental note that Sarah needed a pretty extensive dressing change sometime in the morning. Since Sarah was on contact isolation precautions due to the staph infection, Vickie decided to go ahead and gather all of the dressing change supplies, as well as the supplies that she needed to administer the antibiotic. This would save a tremendous amount of time. With her arms loaded with supplies, Vickie walked down the hallway into Sarah's room. She put on her paper gown and latex-free gloves prior to entering Sarah's room. This decreased the risk of spreading staph infection to the other patients. Upon entering the room, Vickie placed the dressing change supplies on the nightstand and explained to Sarah that she would come back later to complete her dressing change.

Then, following verification that she had the right patient, right medication, right dose, right time, right route, and acknowledging the patient's right to refuse, Vickie scanned the barcode on the medication and on Sarah's arm band. The computer confirmed that Sarah was in fact the patient that was supposed to receive that dosage of medication at that particular time. So Vickie hung the IV antibiotic at 8:10 a.m. and documented that she did so. Vickie noted that it would take approximately one hour for the medication to infuse. The hour would give her time to administer her other patients' morning medications and complete Mr. Smith's discharge.

The only patient whom Vickie had not seen by 8:20 a.m. was Mr. Smith. She knew that she would need to offer him her undivided attention and provide a tremendous amount of education and support before his discharge. Thus, she had waited to complete his assessment after her other patients. She verified and gathered all of Mr. Smith's morning medications, as well as his discharge paperwork. After she informed the nursing assistant and the charge nurse of where she would be for at least 30 minutes, she was off to Mr. Smith's room. First, following a brief physical assessment, she administered Mr. Smith's medications as she verbalized the name of them and explained their purpose. Second, she sat down in a chair next to Mr. Smith's bed. Vickie was experienced in asking the right questions at the right time — questions that got to the heart of an issue. She used the same methods that Jesus used throughout His life on earth.

Mr. Smith acknowledged that the social worker had visited with him regarding housing, food, and medication assistance programs, and that the social worker "seemed like she was going to try to help." Vickie affirmed that his health and quality of life would be greatly benefited by these programs. He nodded his understanding. After about 20 minutes of offering Mr. Smith some tips on managing his health with little-to-no financial provisions, Vickie had him sign his discharge papers, and ensured that he had the appropriate contact information in tow. The social worker had arranged for public transportation to be awaiting Mr. Smith upon discharge to take him to the local homeless shelter. Mr. Smith had agreed. Vickie shook his hand, wished him well, and went back to the nurses' station to check the computer for any new or pending providers' orders.

When Vickie looked at Mr. Hill's chart, she noticed that the doctor had ordered two units of packed red blood cells to be infused immediately following his colonoscopy. This confirmed Vickie's earlier prediction. She quickly made a note in bright red in Mr. Hill's section of her report sheet and asked the nursing assistant to alert her as soon as Mr. Hill arrived back on the unit. The nursing assistant agreed. Vickie went on to successfully care for all of her patients that day, and even admitted two more while on her shift without becoming overwhelmed. Her patients felt that they had been loved and cared for by a competent, effective, efficient, organized nurse.

Without careful organization, Vickie's day could have become a chaotic disaster in a hurry. Disorganization has the potential to jeopardize patients' lives and the quality of care which they receive. There will always be unexpected events and nuances that no one can anticipate. However, arriving early, mentally and spiritually preparing for the day, keeping organized records, prioritizing care, and utilizing appropriate delegation are a few of the many ways that nurses can improve the lives of patients and remain competent in the care they provide.

If you are not an organized person, please do not fret. Unlike compassion, organization can be taught and learned. Over the next several days, I challenge you think of the most successful, organized people in your life. Observe them, ask them how they anticipate, plan, and execute day-to-day and moment-to-moment activities. Then, examine your own life. Determine what areas could use improved organization. Do you need to start writing things in a planner or putting reminders in your phone? Perhaps you are already an organized person and do not need assistance in this area. If so, congratulations! You are one step closer to becoming a successful, efficient, effective nurse. However, if you find yourself feeling overwhelmed at the thought of juggling five patients, take a deep breath and relax. Know that there are people out there who will be more than willing to help you on this journey. As a nursing professor, I have assisted many students to overcome extreme disorganization. All you need is a willing heart and a teachable spirit.

My Prayer for You

Heavenly Father,

You are a God of order. From the beginning of time, You executed things with great organization. You created the heavens, the earth, and all of life without any sign of chaos. The earth continues to rotate around the sun, day-by-day and season-by-season. I praise You for Your organization and that not one sparrow will fall to the ground outside of Your will. Thank You for Jesus' example of how to ask relevant, deep, loving questions that penetrate directly to the heart. Father, please bless the person reading this book with mentors who can model heavenly order and organization before them. Allow them to be teachable and willing to learn from those with wisdom and experience. Give them the ability to ask questions as Jesus did, in order to utilize their time wisely and to quickly see into the heart of another.

In Jesus' Holy and most precious name, Amen.

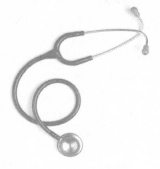

Chapter 11

A Firm Foundation: Curriculum Choices

Would you ever build your home on a foundation made of sand? I doubt it! A home constructed on a foundation made of sand would slip into the sea when the waves crashed against the shore. Would you build your home on a foundation made of wood? I assume, again, your answer would be "no." A home built on a wooden foundation would eventually rot and collapse after years of wear and tear. What would your response be if someone asked you if you would desire a marriage built on a foundation of lies and deceit? A resounding "NO" again, I'm sure. A marriage built on a foundation of lies would surely end badly. Foundations are vital in the development and stability of anything. If a foundation is not firm and secure, the structure or concept built upon it is doomed. Foundations must be strong and virtually indestructible.

Think about a rock. How difficult is it to destroy a rock? When you throw a rock, it doesn't shatter like glass and rarely even chips or cracks. In the Ozark Mountains, it requires strong men with industrial equipment and dynamite to blast through the rock in order to construct interstates and highways. I don't know about you, but I would like my house built upon a rock foundation. Jesus said that a wise man builds his house upon the rock. So when the rains fall, the floods come, and the winds beat upon the house, it will not fall because of its strong foundation. Likewise, He said that a foolish man builds his house upon the sand. So, when the rains fall, the floods come, and the winds beat upon the house, it would definitely experience a great fall. This was a metaphor that Jesus used to explain the consequences of hearing His words and choosing not to obey them (Matthew 7:24–27).

Just as your relationship with Jesus Christ is the rock-solid foundation in which to establish your life, nurses must have a rock-solid foundation, including sound curriculum choices, on which to build their professional careers. When the majority of individuals are asked the most important components of curriculum choices for nurses, they will typically respond with science and math. Don't get me wrong, a sound understanding of science and mathematics is essential in the profession of nursing. As a young naïve nurse, I frequently stated that my patients did not care whether I knew that Columbus sailed the ocean blue in 1492, or that I could speak in perfect, grammatically correct sentences, but more so whether I knew what was going on in their bodies and could efficiently and correctly mathematically calculate their medication dosages. (You must know that I am a southern girl with a thick southern accent. Unfortunately, we southerners are often accused of speaking unintelligently and adding extra syllables to our words. I cannot deny the syllable accusation, but unintelligent, I think not!)

However, as I have grown in the profession of nursing and as a believer in the Body of Christ, I have learned that although math and science are critical curriculum choices, reading comprehension and the ability to communicate effectively, think critically, and reason clinically are of equal or even superior importance. Statistics positively support the relationship between these qualities and increased NCLEX-RN[1] success.[2] That's good news, especially since children usually start communicating at birth and learn to read in kindergarten! Think about how many years a person has to perfect these abilities. So the next time you start to groan about taking the ACT or SAT, remember that the foundational concepts that these tests are designed to examine are only helping you along your journey to becoming a successful nurse.

Becoming a successful nurse requires wise curriculum choices long before you even enter college. Don't worry. Most of your junior high and high school curriculums are designed to set you up for success in any field of study. This is because they are well rounded. You must complete courses in math, science, English, literature, and history. However, when you enter college, you have the freedom to choose the courses in which you would like to enroll. This can become overwhelming, but your college advisor (someone who is assigned to you based on your major) will assist you in this endeavor.

Schools and colleges of nursing are governed by various certifying bodies and state boards of nursing with regard to curriculum design. They are required to include specific courses in various areas of study based upon the level of degree which they offer. For example, students completing a Bachelor of Science in Nursing degree must successfully complete prerequisite courses including anatomy, physiology, chemistry, psychology or sociology, English, history, etc. Although nurses must possess knowledge of anatomy, physiology, and pathophysiology, they also must have the ability to solve relatively difficult algebraic

---

1. National Council Licensure Examination for RNs.
2. A.O. Arhin and E. Cormier, "Using Deconstruction to Educate Generation Y Nursing Students," *Educational Innovations*, December 2007, 46(12), 562–567.

equations when calculating medication dosages and IV drip rates. Again, these are all extremely important in nursing. But let's think about a nurse who possesses these skills and abilities, but cannot comprehend a patient's chart, lacks the ability to critically think through a sudden change in a patient's condition, fails miserably at clinically reasoning the next most appropriate nursing intervention, and possesses the communication skills of a brick wall. That does not sound like a nurse that I would like to have caring for me or someone I love.

So how does one become an effectively communicating, critically thinking, clinically reasoning, successful nurse? The answer is not black and white, but more one of a gray hue. It starts with an open mind and a willing heart. Before you go into convulsions when the nursing curriculum in which you enroll requires you to take public speaking, think deeply about how a nurse must be able to effectively communicate with patients, families, and other members of the healthcare team. Public speaking courses rank highest on most of my students' complaint lists. However, these courses build confidence, enhance communication skills, and assist individuals in succinctly and successfully getting a point across. In the age of texting, instant messaging, and social media, people have forgotten how to have a conversation. News flash! Texting a patient who is actively vomiting about the medication you are administering into their IV is probably not advisable. Conversation is mandatory!

Not only is conversation mandatory in nursing, but so is critical thinking. I think I have mentioned that a time or two. Perhaps you are already an astute critical thinker or maybe you are asking yourself exactly what I mean by critical thinking. I will err on the side of caution and explain critical thinking in the context of nursing. To critically think in nursing is to examine an entire situation, the whole picture, including subjective and objective data, and then differentiate the relevant from the irrelevant. I like the way that Scripture says to "take forth the precious from the vile" (Jeremiah 15:19; KJV). In a sense, that is what a nurse must do when assessing and analyzing a patient's situation.

A nurse must approach a situation and critically think while considering his or her own biases and examining any assumptions that he or she may have regarding the situation. Let's see what this looks like when applied to a clinical situation. You are the nurse caring for a 17-year-old female patient with sudden onset right lower abdominal pain accompanied by nausea and vomiting. She was brought to the hospital by a young man who appears to be her age. Her hair is disheveled and her clothes are wrinkled, and her body is covered with tattoos and piercings. Now, let's examine the hard evidence.

First, subjectively, your patient is 17 years old and complaining of right lower abdominal pain and nausea. Second, objectively, you visualize that your patient is a female who is vomiting, cringing, and holding her abdomen, with unkempt hair and clothes, has multiple tattoos and piercings, and is accompanied by a young male. At this point, you must sort through the information we have gathered and only focus on what is valuable, relevant, and necessary to provide appropriate nursing care. You must separate the "precious" from the "vile."

Before you do this, ask yourself if you have any biases with regard to this patient or situation. Perhaps you think that it is wrong for a man and woman to live together prior to marriage. If this is the case, you may have the assumption that your patient is promiscuous, the young man who brought your patient to the hospital is her boyfriend, and that her pain is related to pregnancy. Your bias may have led you to the wrong assumption. Perhaps the young man with your patient is her brother. He may have transported her to the hospital because they both recently lost their parents in a fatal car accident, and he is the only person she has in her support system at this time. Another potential assumption could be that your patient is poor and immature since she is 17 and came to the hospital in unlaundered, wrinkled clothes. However, your assumption may be incorrect again. Maybe it was late at night when your patient's pain started and she just came to the hospital in the clothes she wore to bed. Be very cautious of biases and assumptions. They can hinder your nursing care and dim your reflection of the light of Jesus to your patients.

Take a moment and go back to the subjective and objective evidence that you gathered in the initial assessment. What information is relevant to your patient's diagnosis and treatment? What information is of no significance? A nurse equipped with the skill of critical thinking would note that the patient is a young female with sudden onset of right lower abdominal pain. A prudent nurse might consider that the patient's pain could be related to pregnancy, but would not make that assumption until more information is gathered. Since you are a prudent nurse that examined your own biases and put them aside, as well as eliminated any assumptions that could mask the real issue, you begin to ask relevant poignant questions so that you can clinically reason through the situation. "Have you ever experienced this pain before?" "Can you describe what the pain feels like (sharp, dull, aching)?" "Does the pain radiate or remain in one spot?" "Have you ever had surgery to remove your appendix?" These are only a few questions that a critically thinking nurse would ask. After several unbiased, relevant questions, a critically thinking nurse would, again, sift through and synthesize the newly gathered information.

Once all patient information has been gathered, analyzed, and synthesized, and sorted according to relevancy, a nurse must move into clinical reasoning. Critical thinking is sometimes used interchangeably with clinical reasoning. However, they are actually related concepts that just happen to mesh well together. A professional nurse must possess both. Clinical reasoning involves examination of gathered evidence, determination of issues/problems, creation of goals, and conclusion of appropriate nursing interventions.

For example, the nurse equipped with the ability to clinically reason would listen to each of the patient's responses to the questions asked. He or she would group related things together: sudden onset pain; located in the right lower quadrant; no history of appendix removal; recent major increase in stress. Then the nurse might determine that the patient is suffering from appendicitis. This is obviously a medical diagnosis and a problem that requires surgical intervention. However, until the surgeon arrives, the nurse should address the major problems the patient is facing, such as pain and emotional distress. Often, if a person's pain is addressed, other issues such as anxiety will subside. At this point, a clinically reasoning nurse would visit with the patient about acceptable levels of pain and set mutually acceptable goals. Then the nurse would medicate the patient for pain and offer non-pharmacological interventions, such as music therapy, distraction, and various environmental alterations (dim lighting, cool room). Once the nurse completes the interventions, the patient would require re-assessment or evaluation to determine if the interventions were successful or not. If they were, then the same plan could be continued. However, if they were not successful, the nurse and the patient would need to re-examine their goals to make sure that they were reasonable and appropriate.

You may be saying to yourself that the attributes of effective communication, critical thinking, and sound, clinical reasoning seem easy. If so, fantastic! In order to have a rock-solid foundation for developing and maintaining a nurse of excellence, these attributes are vital. They do, however, require hard work, practice, and dedication. In the profession of nursing, learning never ceases. There are constantly new and innovative skills, procedures, and medications being developed throughout healthcare that nurses have to continuously hone and sharpen. This chapter is simply an overview of the curricular foundation for nursing. In order to remain successful, nurses must not only have a strong foundation, but must also be willing to continue to build on their foundation for years to come.

My Prayer for You

Heavenly Father,

You are the foundation of the world. Without You, the solar system would collapse; gravity would cease to keep things in perfect motion; the earth would not rotate around the sun; there would be no day or night; our lives would be chaos. So, Father, I thank You and praise You for Your intelligent creation of this earth and all that is within it. Thank You for the firm foundation of Your Holy Scripture. I praise You for instilling the necessities of sound curricular design in nursing to those who have gone before me. I pray that the person reading this book will view the foundational curriculum for nursing as vital and necessary. Furthermore, I pray that they will complete each course, whether it is science, math, or public speaking, as a form of worship unto You. Please provide them with strength and perseverance as they journey along this most incredibly blessed career path to nursing.

In Jesus' Holy and most precious name, Amen.

Chapter 12

The Temperature of Nursing: A Range of Degrees

You have probably heard the saying, "There is more than one way to skin a cat." Well, in anatomy and physiology lab, you may quickly find that this is true. Nursing could easily adopt a similar slogan: "There is more than one way to become a nurse." There are a multitude of levels of nursing and various degrees which one can attain within the profession. It is easy to visualize the levels and ranges of degrees when compared to body temperature. Although 98.6 degrees Fahrenheit is considered the ideal core body temperature, there is a significant range of temperatures that are acceptable and healthy. Nurses range from licensed practical to doctorally prepared — each of which is important and valuable.

Although not classified or referred to as "nurses," certified nursing assistants (CNAs) are very much a vital part of the nursing team. CNAs are considered frontline healthcare workers. They work alongside and under the direction of nurses to ensure optimal care, providing the majority of basic care for hospital patients, nursing home residents, and patients in the community setting.

This includes bathing, toileting, transferring, and assisting with other activities of daily living. CNAs also spend a significant amount of time listening, consoling, and comforting those in their care. In order to become a CNA, one must complete two weeks or 75 contact hours of training and pass a certification examination.[1]

Licensed practical or licensed vocational nurses (LPN/LVN) are also vital members of the nursing team and work alongside CNAs and other nurses to provide effective quality care. LPN and LVN programs must be state approved, and take approximately one year to complete.[2] In order to obtain licensure, LPN/LVNs must successfully complete the National Council Licensure Examination for Licensed Practical/Vocational Nurses (NCLEX-PN). The LPN/LVN scope of practice varies from state-to-state. However, LPN/LVNs must practice under the direction of registered professional nurses. In the majority of states within the United States, LPNs/LVNs can provide basic care (activities of daily living), offer non-pharmacological (heat and cold therapy, massage, positioning, etc.) therapies to increase comfort, and are qualified to administer oral medications and a multitude of injections, not including intravenous injections or blood transfusions; although a variety of states recognize intravenous certifications for LPNs/LVNs. Many state practice acts also mandate that LPN/LVNs cannot perform comprehensive assessments,[3] and there is significant variability among states with regard to LPN/LVNs and nursing assessment, care planning,

---

1. Institute of Medicine, *Retooling for an Aging America: Building the Health-care Workforce* (Washington DC: National Academies Press, 2008).

2. Bureau of Labor Statistics, U.S. Department of Labor, Occupational Outlook Handbook, 2014–15 Edition, Registered Nurses, http://www.bls.gov/ooh/healthcare/registered-nurses.htm.

3. K.N. Corazzini, R.A. Anderson, C. Mueller, E.S. McConnell, L.R. Landerman, J.M. Thorpe, N.M. Short, "Regulation of LPN Scope of Practice in Long-term Care," *Journal of Nursing Regulation*, 2011, 2(2), 30–36.

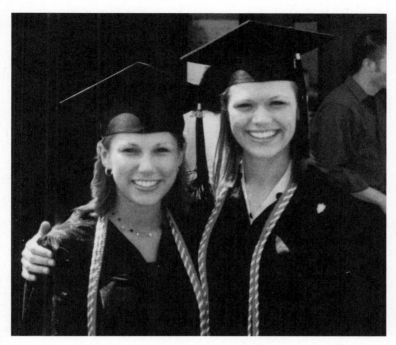

My cousin Jaye Henderson and me at BSN graduation

delegation, and supervision.[4] Nonetheless, LPN/LVNs play an important role within the profession, with approximately 70 percent of licensed care provided in nursing care facilities being fulfilled by this population.[5]

Another group of valuable members of the nursing team include registered nurses (RN). RNs not only provide patient care, but they also coordinate care and provide education to patients and the public about health promotion and illness

---

4. National League for Nursing Board of Governors, "A Vision for Recognition of the Role of Licensed Practical/Vocational Nurses in Advancing the Nation's Health," *NLN Vision Series*, September 2014, 1–7, http://www. nln.org/aboutnln/livingdocuments/pdf/nlnvision_7.pdf.

5. Corazzini et al., "Regulation of LPN Scope of Practice in Long-term Care."

prevention.[6] RNs can work in virtually any setting: hospitals, nursing care facilities, schools, the military, prisons, and the list is practically endless. RNs can either earn an associate's degree or a bachelor's degree. Associate Degree in Nursing (ADN) programs are typically two to three years in length, whereas Bachelor of Science in Nursing (BSN) degree programs take approximately four years to complete. The BSN prepared nurse receives additional education in critical thinking, leadership, and management; therapeutic and professional communication; as well as the physical and social sciences. This additional education prepares the BSN-RN for administrative, teaching, research, and consulting positions.[7]

Individuals desiring to further their education and work in advanced practice positions have the opportunity to obtain advanced degrees, such as a Master of Science in Nursing (MSN), a Doctor of Nursing Practice (DNP), and/or a Doctor of Philosophy (PhD) degree. There are a variety of different options in which nurses can earn these degrees. A nurse can opt for the traditional route, beginning with a BSN degree, advancing to a MSN degree, and then completing either a DNP or PhD as their terminal degree. However, this route is not always feasible for everyone, especially those with children, single parents, single-income households, etc. Therefore, many nursing programs across the United States offer "bridge" programs. These are accelerated programs that allow individuals with some level of nursing degree, or even a degree in another profession, to cross over a hypothetical "bridge" to a higher nursing degree. This can include LPN-to-ADN bridges, ADN-to-BSN bridges, ADN-to-MSN bridges, BSN-to-DNP bridges, and the list continues.

---

6. Bureau of Labor Statistics, U.S. Department of Labor, Occupational Outlook Handbook, 2014–15 Edition, Registered Nurses, http://www.bls.gov/ooh/healthcare/registered-nurses.htm.

7. Ibid.

Typically, when one refers to an "advanced" nursing degree, they mean a MSN or beyond. These degrees open up a multitude of opportunities for nurses. The master's or doctorally prepared nurse can specialize in several different areas: family, pediatric, geriatric, adult, or acute care nurse practitioner; nurse midwife; certified registered nurse anesthetist; and nurse educator, just to name a few.

Nurse practitioners are considered mid-level providers and can see patients in the hospital, nursing home, clinic, or community settings. Their scope of practice varies from state to state, but generally, nurse practitioners can assess, diagnose, and devise treatment plans (including prescribing medications) in the majority of states within the United States.

Nurse midwives can provide pre-, ante-, and post-natal care for women, as well as deliver babies. Certified registered nurse anesthetists administer anesthesia and monitor patients before, during, and after surgery. In the majority of states, these advanced practice specialty nurses work in collaboration with physicians who also practice within their selected specialty. Although I could write forever about nursing education, I assume that the nurse educator requires no further explanation.

In conclusion, you can deduce that nursing is a profession full of options and choices just waiting to be considered. No matter the specialty chosen, nurses are all special. No matter the degree obtained, the temperature of nursing has a variety of healthy ranges. No matter the road traveled in order to obtain the degree, the road to nursing is sacred. No matter the patient population for which a nurse cares, people are human beings created in the image of God. What will your choice be? What degree will you strive to achieve? What road will you travel to arrive there? No matter your response to these questions, nursing requires passion, drive, motivation, perseverance, understanding, compassion, empathy, and, most of all, love. Without these, the temperature of nursing falls outside of a healthy range and is not sustainable to life.

My Prayer for You

Heavenly Father,

Thank You so much for designing the human body to be resilient with a range of healthy temperatures. Thank You for providing nurses with such a magnitude of options for degrees and specialties, and a plethora of healthy avenues in which to travel there. What an incredible profession! I am so grateful that You called me to be a nurse. I pray that the person reading this book recognizes, realizes, and understands that You have plans for them, plans to give them a hope and a future. If that future is in nursing, I pray that they will allow You to guide them in choosing the degree, specialty, and avenue that leads to a temperature that remains healthy throughout their lifetime.

In Jesus' Holy and most precious name, Amen.

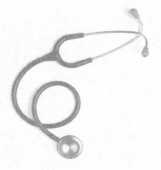

Chapter 13

Endless Opportunities

The thought of doing the same, repetitious action day in and day out, thousands of times per day literally makes me cringe. Don't get me wrong — there is absolutely nothing wrong with working on an assembly line in a factory or adding numbers in an accounting office all day. Without people in those positions, the world could not go around. However, those jobs require frequent repetition and offer little opportunity for creativity. I like to think of myself as a more adventurous person, someone who enjoys a challenge and embraces change. This is probably why God called me to be a nurse.

A nursing career affords a person a multitude of opportunities. In fact, the opportunities are virtually endless. First of all, human beings are extremely complicated. We are the most complicated living beings on earth. Not only do we possess physical bodies that are constantly growing, developing, aging, and changing, but we also have complicated emotional and spiritual components that require much attention, tender love, and care. Nurses must be prepared to offer this complex, multifaceted, ever-changing care.

Over the years, several have made the claim that "nurses wear many hats." Metaphorically speaking, this is the truth. As you have already read in previous chapters, a nurse may be performing chest compressions on a child one minute and holding the hands of a dying older adult the next. A nurse is one of the few professions that counsels, teaches, mothers, leads, calms, comforts, holds, medicates, bathes, and saves the lives of others. And this is just a short list!

Not only do nurses perform all of these duties, but we complete them around the clock, in a variety of locations, on a host of different people. So, you have an extreme disdain for mornings, and the average cup of coffee just does not do the job. That is not a problem if you are a nurse. You have options! Nurses can work part-time, full-time, weekends, or as needed (PRN). Nursing shifts in the hospital vary from 8 hours to 12 hours per day, and can be day, evening, or night shift. It is up to the nurse to choose what is best for his or her life.

Not only do nurses have the option to choose what shift we prefer to work, but we can also choose from a variety of different locations in which we would like to be employed. By location, I don't simply mean geographic location, such as urban or rural, national or international. The great news is that location also includes the physical building in which a nurse works. This could be in a hospital (inpatient or outpatient), clinic, rehabilitation facility, nursing home, school, a patient's home, a camp, a village, or even a prison. The list has the potential to continue forever. And, to compound the great news, nurses can change job location or setting at any time during their careers. If we get tired or bored or maybe burned out, we can change locations, settings, or positions to add a little spice.

Maybe you are like I was and are not sure in which location or setting you wish to work. During nursing school, it is almost like a buffet of choices. Nursing school affords you the opportunity to peruse both sides of the buffet, sampling a variety of different work settings for short bursts of time. For example, when I began my BSN degree, I thought I wanted to work in pediatrics. My, how that changed! I now work as a professor teaching geriatrics and adult care. So do not get frustrated when you cannot decide what particular aspect of nursing interests you. That will come, and trust me, it will change.

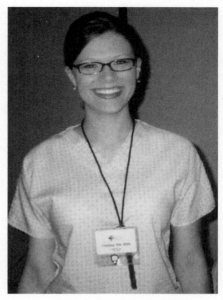

My first day as an RN at Skaggs Community Hospital

Perhaps you start off working in a hospital as an emergency room nurse. The adrenaline rush gets you excited and you love the invigoration that comes over your body when you are involved in saving the life of a patient who has experienced a traumatic accident. Then, maybe a year or so down the road, you decide that you have had enough adrenaline and want to experience something a little mellower. You could work as a nurse in an outpatient women's health clinic, providing education to women of all ages about how to achieve and maintain optimal health.

Two years later, the desire for adrenaline may return and you could enlist in the military and serve your country as a military nurse. This might include working in a veteran's hospital or literally on the frontlines of the battlefield. You might be saying to yourself, bullets and limb loss may be a bit overwhelming for an extended period of time. If so, how about serving precious tiny babies and their families in a neonatal intensive care unit? Some babies in these units are one pound! Yes, I said ONE pound. In fact, two of my nephews and one of my nieces weighed barely over one pound each at birth. If it had not been for their phenomenal nurses, they may not be here with us today. What an honor and privilege to serve as a nurse in this capacity!

However, maybe tiny babies scare you and you would rather work in a nursing home serving the older adult population. The wisdom that they have to offer and the deep appreciation for your service may motivate you to continue nursing with excellence. Or, maybe, just maybe, you like instant gratification and want to see the fruit of your labor right away. The operating room may be a great place for you. Assisting in the removal of a large cancerous tumor and knowing that a patient is now cancer-free, may bring you great joy.

At this point, you might be saying to yourself, "All I really want to do is travel. Where can I find a job that allows me to do that?" Look no further! Nursing also affords you great travel opportunities. After a few years of experience, a nurse can sign up with a travel agency and work several weeks in one location, then the next several weeks in another location. If your favorite pastime is lying on the beach feeling the warmth of the sun beaming down on your face, Hawaii or Florida may be the location you choose to land. Or maybe you prefer snuggling up by the fire with a good book after a day of snow skiing. Then you may want to work in the mountains of Colorado. This, too, is a possibility. The travel agencies pay your salary, provide you with a place to live, and give you per diem monies for eating and entertainment. Hefty sign-on and completion bonuses are not unusual with these agencies either.

But if Hawaii, Florida, or Colorado is not adventurous enough for you, maybe working on the mission field in a village in Africa or the jungles of Ecuador would better fulfill your desires. I have nursing graduates in both locations, and the stories they share with me are virtually unbelievable. When doctors, surgeons, and hospital facilities are hours away from villages and jungles, these nurses do what is life saving and necessary. This may include temporarily suturing a laceration by allowing large ants to bite along the length of the cut, pinching the ant bodies off and leaving their heads in place to stop the bleeding and hold the cut together until more contemporary measures can be taken.

Adventurous, hands-on nursing is not for everyone. Maybe you would rather be a nurse of inquiry and discovery. There are nurses who work solely in research, creating "best practice" standards for others to follow; nurses who speak to other nurses to motivate and inspire; nurses who work for insurance agencies ensuring beneficiaries are receiving the most appropriate interventions; nurses who work for medication manufacturers and consult with pharmacies and prescribers; nurses who lead and manage hospital units or entire organizations; advanced practice nurses who fill in the primary care gaps when serving the minor acutely ill population; nurses who invent, design, and develop products to assist others in their journey to health; nurses who write books and research articles to disseminate the most relevant, evidence-based practice guidelines; nurses who teach in hospitals or colleges working diligently to cultivate new nurses and continue this great profession.

Nurses can virtually do anything and go anywhere. This chapter just touches the tip of the iceberg of opportunities within nursing. The opportunities truly are endless. However, we must keep in mind, "The heart of man plans his way, but the LORD establishes his steps" (Proverbs 16:9). This is certainly something that I have learned throughout my career of many changes. Nonetheless, I am excited and encouraged to know that, even after ten years in the profession of nursing, my heart is still full and continuously ready to see what is awaiting me around the next corner.

My Prayer for You

Heavenly Father,

Wow! Thank You so much for a career that is exciting, invigorating, ever-changing, never boring, and always rewarding. My heart overflows with joy in knowing that You have called me to such an amazing career filled with opportunity. I pray that the person reading this book will be inspired by this chapter. I pray that You open their hearts and minds to the possibilities that await them. Let them dream, and dream big! Remind them that You allow them to have desires, but that, ultimately, You plan their steps. Comfort them with the understanding that Your plan is far better than any dream or ideal they can imagine. Thank You, Father, for loving us so much and allowing us to love others through the great profession of nursing.

In Jesus' Holy and most precious name, Amen.

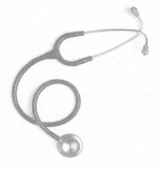

Chapter 14

It's More
Than Salary

More money . . . a bigger house . . . a nicer car . . . wouldn't we all love to have more money, a bigger house, and a nicer car!? Contrary to popular conservative belief, none of these things are bad. However, the *love* of them can most certainly cause a person to venture down the road to destruction. First Timothy 6:10 says that, "For the love of money is a root of all kinds of evils." Houses and cars are temporary earthly treasures that begin to depreciate almost simultaneously with the moment of purchase, and money is only as valuable as the market deems it. Don't get me wrong, it would not hurt my feelings to have a little higher salary, an extra bedroom and bathroom in my home, and a larger, more luxurious vehicle. However, the Lord says,

> Do not lay up for yourselves treasures on earth, where moth and rust destroy and where thieves break in and steal (Matthew 6:19).

Wow! Moths and rust do destroy. Might I add that mice do too? Some of my best clothes have become the diet and beds of the mice that creep in through the crevices of our little log cabin built in 1930. And rust — don't get me started on rust. Living in the Midwest, we often have unpredictable icy, snowy, slushy winter weather. Our highway department is phenomenal and keeps the roads salted three to four months out of the year. Although the roads are safer, secondary to this our cars sadly suffer the consequences. So, fancy clothes and luxurious vehicles may seem like worthy investments, but I try to remind myself that they are temporary. Temporary until moth, mice, or rust destroy, or temporary until Christ returns and calls us home.

Thinking about earthly treasures in this manner assuredly changed my perspective, as I hope it does yours, too. Most people in America live to work and work to live. It is like the never-ending hamster wheel. We work diligently day in and day out to put more money in our retirement fund, save to go on a vacation that rarely occurs, and to earn enough to leave an inheritance to our loved ones when we die. But why? Do any of these things impart true joy in our hearts or fulfill our deepest desires? Let me answer that for you — "NO!" Perhaps they do bring us moments of temporary pleasure, but once the new is worn off, the vacation is over, or the market crashes, the contentment ceases, and it is right back to the hamster wheel.

The good news is that nurses do not have to remain on the hamster wheel. We have the honor and privilege to "lay up for [ourselves] treasures in heaven, where neither moth nor rust destroys and where thieves do not break in and steal" (Matthew 6:20). In reality, every individual on earth is afforded this opportunity. Nurses just have a unique environment in which to do so. The people for whom nurses provide care are in some of the most vulnerable states in life. To assist in alleviating someone's pain, holding another's hand so they do not have to die alone, or leading a patient in the prayer of salvation are undoubtedly heavenly treasures that no one or nothing can steal or destroy.

Praise God for this daily opportunity to serve others and accumulate heavenly treasures! Nonetheless, nurses still have to earn a living to survive in the hamster wheel of life and work. The great news is that the nursing profession has the ability to provide job security and a stable, comfortable income. First, as many factories, retail stores, and small businesses are being forced to shut their doors, hospitals, clinics, and nursing homes do not face this same sort of danger. Populations continue to grow. People are living longer. And the human body is continuously "wasting away" (2 Corinthians 4:16). Therefore, there will always be a need for nurses to provide care for the sick and hurting.

From 2008 to 2010, there were approximately 2,824,641 RNs and 690,038 LPNs working within the nursing profession across the United States.[1] The Bureau of Labor Statistics anticipates a 19.4 percent increase in job openings by 2022. That is equivalent to 526,800 new jobs, supporting the stability and security of working in this great profession. When many organizations are replacing people with computers and robotic machines, nurses can relax. Robots do not have the ability to critically think, let alone demonstrate compassion — two vital components in nursing.

Speaking of robots and technology . . . the world is becoming increasingly obsessed and dependent on computers and technology. This is lending to the rising cost of vehicles, cell phones, and all of the other techie gadgets, such as tablets and iPads. The rising cost of goods and services inevitably induces higher costs of living. In 1982 (the year I was born), the average annual income in the United States of America was $14,531.34. The average income across all employed Americans in 2013 was $44,888.16, indicative of a $10,000 annual rise in income.[2]

---

1. U.S. Dept. of Health and Human Services, http://bhpr.hrsa.gov/.

2. http://www.ssa.gov/oact/cola/AWI.html.

This seems likes a sizeable increase, but is it really? The average cost of a two-bedroom home in 1982 was only $83,900. However, by 2014, it skyrocketed to over $350,000.[3] That's nearly a 420 percent increase in only 32 years!

So how are nursing salaries keeping up with inflation and the ever-increasing price tags associated with the United States' cost of living? Over the last ten years, full-time (36 hours or more per week) RN salaries have increased approximately $20,000 and LPN salaries have increased approximately $11,500.[4] The median annual salary of an RN in 2013 was $66,220, with the highest-paid RNs earning more than $90,000 per year. Even the lowest paid RNs made around $45,000 annually,[5] still slightly higher than the average income of all other professions.

Earning potential for nurses does not stop with registered or licensed practical nurse title attainment. Level of experience; working weekends, evenings, or nights; earning certifications in various specialty areas; and obtaining advanced nursing degrees all come with higher paychecks. For example, nurse practitioners have an average annual salary of approximately $95,070,[6] whereas certified registered nurse anesthetists can earn upwards of $150,000 to $220,000 per year.[7] And these statistics are just average and median salaries, simply brushing the tip of the iceberg of a nurse's earning potential. There is insurance, retirement, and a multitude of additional benefits afforded to those entering the nursing profession.

Benefits and comfortable salaries may sound appealing and amplify your interest in committing to a lifetime of serving

3. www.census.gov.
4. U.S. Dept. of Health and Human Services, http://bhpr.hrsa.gov/.
5. Bureau of Labor Statistics, http://www.bls.gov/.
6. U.S. News and World Report, http://money.usnews.com/careers/best-jobs/nurse-practitioner/salary.
7. Bureau of Labor Statistics, http://www.bls.gov/.

others through the profession of nursing. However, again, these are earthly treasures. Sure, they make life a little easier and more comfortable, but they are material things that moths and rust can destroy and thieves can break in and steal. Let me express to you that nursing is much more than salary. Words cannot captivate the overwhelming satisfaction a nurse experiences when a mother says, "Thank you for saving my child," or the warmth that floods the body when a nurse receives a card offering words of gratitude for holding the hand of a dying mother when the daughter could not be there, or the emotional delight experienced from a patient's embrace for care they received from a nurse decades earlier. Encounters such as these are heavenly treasures — those that nothing can destroy and no one can steal, for it is impossible to ruin or burglarize unconditional love and compassion.

My Prayer for You

Heavenly Father,

Thank You so much for affording nurses the opportunity to earn a comfortable, secure living. Thank You for the earthly treasures that my career in nursing has always made possible: maintaining a roof over my head, food on my table, and clothes on my back. But more than that, thank You for the heavenly treasures that this amazing career has provided me: the decade of memories shared with my patients and their families; the tears of sadness and joy that have come from loving and caring so deeply for others; the wisdom imparted to me from those entrusted in my care; the numerous cards, letters, and gifts that emanated gratitude far better than any amount of money; and the excitement and enthusiasm I feel every day that I get to be a nurse. I pray that the person reading this book now understands that nursing is much more than salary. I pray that at the conclusion of their nursing career, their heavenly treasure far outweighs their earthly treasure.

In Jesus' Holy and most precious name, Amen.

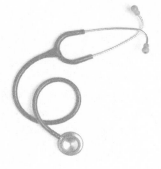

Chapter 15

Nursing Process: Just AD-PIE

There is a process for just about everything that we do in life. Some processes may have more ingredients or steps, and be much lengthier than others, but nonetheless, are still processes. The process of pasteurizing milk includes heating one ingredient or raw substance, the milk, to a certain temperature for seconds to minutes. Although it includes only one main ingredient, sugar cane, the process of refining sugar is much longer and encompasses over 25 different steps. Making a pie includes several ingredients, and the time from initiation to completion varies depending upon the type of pie. The process of fetal development in a mother's womb encompasses millions of cells and the miraculous process transpires over 40 weeks! If an ingredient is forgotten, a step is omitted, or the appropriate length of time is not heeded, the end product of these processes would be less than ideal.

The profession of nursing also has a process that requires careful consideration in order to best care for patients. In order to not forget an ingredient or omit a step, utilization of the acronym AD-PIE is extremely valuable. This process offers structure and standardization in the way that nurses provide patient care. It strengthens quality, effectiveness, and efficiency. AD-PIE stands for: (A) Assessment; (D) Diagnosis; (P) Plan; (I) Implementation; and (E) Evaluation.

Nursing *assessment* is a lot like being an inspector or investigator. It requires incredible scrutiny and discernment, including looking, listening, smelling, and touching. However, tasting is probably not advisable. For example, if a baby is uncontrollably crying, the mother first listens to the tone and quality of the cry. Different cries indicate different needs. She then looks at the infant and notes the color of their skin or whether or not they appear in pain. Furthermore, she touches the child to see if they feel warm, or if their diaper is wet. Lastly, she smells and notes whether or not the baby has soiled itself.

After this thorough assessment, the mother moves on to analyzing and grouping the information that she has just gathered. This is the process of *diagnosing* the problem. For example, imagine the mother hears the baby crying and notices that he or she is rooting and making a suckling noise with his or her mouth. The baby does not appear in pain, its skin is warm, dry, and the color is appropriate to their race. The mother also notes that the baby's diaper is clean and dry without evidence of a foul smell. At this time, the mother groups the crying, rooting, and suckling findings together and diagnoses that the baby must be hungry, especially since the other information that she gathered does not indicate a problem and is unrelated to these assessments.

At this point, the mother has gathered several pieces of assessment data, analyzed the findings, grouped related things together and diagnosed that the baby's problem is hunger. If she stops here and does nothing about the hunger, the baby will continue to cry, becoming increasingly agitated. If the mother fails to feed the child for an extended period of time, the consequences could be detrimental to the baby's health, and even fatal. Therefore, she must proceed to the next step of the process, *planning or outcome identification*. This step can also be equated to *goal setting*. The mother might say to herself, "I want my baby to stop crying as soon as I put the bottle nipple into his or her mouth." One could consider this a reasonable, measurable goal.

Once the goal or outcome has been identified, action must be taken in order to reach the goal. This is completed during the *implementation* phase. The mother goes to the kitchen, washes a bottle, sterilizes a nipple, places the appropriate amount of formula and water or breast milk into the bottle, shakes it, and heats it to a safe temperature. Then she offers the bottle to the baby. She has now completed the implementation phase of the process and moves onto *evaluation*.

During the evaluation phase, the mother determines whether or not her implementations or interventions led to the achievement of her goal or plan. If the baby stops crying and immediately begins sucking on the bottle's nipple, then the mother has correctly assessed, diagnosed, planned, and implemented. She can close the loop and feel confident that she can move onto the next endeavor.

However, if, when the bottle nipple is placed into the baby's mouth, the baby spits it out and continues to cry, the mother would need to re-evaluate the situation. This includes starting over at the assessment phase and trying to determine if there were any clues that she may have missed. Then she either formulates a new diagnosis or confirms that the original diagnosis was correct. If she discovers that the baby is indeed hungry and that her plan is adequate, she may implement new or modified interventions to achieve the goal. This may include trying a different bottle or nipple, changing the temperature of the breast milk or formula, or holding the baby in an alternate position.

The mother would continue this cyclic process until the baby's crying is resolved.

This same process is vital in nursing when providing care for patients. Imagine that you are the nurse caring for Mr. Jones on a medical-surgical nursing unit. Mr. Jones is a 75-year-old Caucasian male who was admitted to the hospital two days ago for pneumonia. You just arrived to assume the care of Mr. Jones. He has been doing well, according to the nurse on the previous shift. However, when you walk into his room to complete his morning assessment, you note that he does not appear to be feeling well at all.

Your *assessment* reveals several objective findings: cool, clammy, pale skin; circumoral cyanosis (bluing around the lips); rapid heart rate; low (85%) oxygen saturation on the monitor (normal is >96%); and crackles in the bases of both lungs. Furthermore, subjectively, Mr. Jones expresses that he has been feeling increasingly short of breath and unable to cough anything up for several hours now. He also states that he is starting to feel "a little dizzy."

You immediately begin analyzing and grouping the assessment findings in order to formulate a nursing *diagnosis*. You realize that shortness of breath, dizziness, pallor, circumoral cyanosis, rapid heart rate, low oxygen saturation, and crackles in the lungs can indicate that Mr. Jones is experiencing a poor exchange of oxygen and carbon dioxide. In relation to all of this evidence, you determine that the appropriate nursing diagnosis is *ineffective gas exchange* related to his disease process (pneumonia). At this point, you know that you must devise a plan and implement it quickly to ensure that Mr. Jones does not continue to decline.

You and Mr. Jones quickly and briefly discuss his plan of care, and mutually agree on the following care plan:

Diagnosis	Plan (Goals/ Outcomes)	Implementation with Rationale
Ineffective Gas Exchange related to disease process (pneumonia) as evidenced by shortness of breath; cool, clammy, pale skin; low oxygen saturation; rapid heart rate; dizziness; and crackles in lungs	(1) Patient's oxygen saturation will increase to greater than 90% within 30 minutes. (2) Patient will deny shortness of breath within 30 minutes.	(1) **Assist patient to a sitting position** (sitting up at 90 degrees or leaning over a table allows for greater lung expansion and improved gas exchange). (2) **Apply oxygen via nasal cannula as prescribed by healthcare provider** (when the lungs are impaired, it is often necessary to supplement oxygen to enhance gas exchange). (3) **Administer rapid-acting inhaled respiratory medications as prescribed by healthcare provider** (inhaled rapid-acting respiratory medications quickly dilate airways to enhance gas exchange). (4) **Encourage patient to cough and deep breathe** (coughing and deep breathing assists in clearing the airway to enhance gas exchange).

You implement one or all of the interventions and then *evaluate* whether or not they are effective in achieving the goals or outcomes in your original plan. If Mr. Jones' oxygen saturation is greater than 90% and he denies shortness of breath in the 30-minute time frame, then your plan worked and you move on to the next highest priority issue that you discover. However, if Mr. Jones' oxygen saturation is only slightly increased to 87%, or perhaps not increased at all, and he is still complaining of shortness of breath within the 30-minute time frame, then you would re-evaluate and modify the care plan. This includes beginning the nursing process over again.

As you can see, following the nursing process when providing patient care is important to maintain order. Instead of blindly approaching and navigating through a situation, the nursing process serves as a roadmap or GPS to assist nurses when caring for patients. In 1 Corinthians chapter 14 there is a lengthy discussion regarding the maintenance of order, even in worship. The chapter is summed up with the words, "But all things should be done decently and in order" (1 Corinthians 14:40). This statement is the truth. Rarely can anything be accomplished in chaos, but when order is maintained, steps are precisely followed, and ingredients are not forgotten . . . products are created, goals are accomplished, and health is restored.

My Prayer for You

Heavenly Father,

Thank You for being a God of order. From the beginning of time, You created and followed a plan. Even in the creation of the heavens and the earth, there was a process. Thank You for leading by example. Thank You for creating us to be creatures designed for order and maintenance. Thank You for providing insight to those who develop processes, such as the nursing process. I pray that I will always be a nurse of order, a nurse who follows the process carefully, and never misses a detail when caring for patients. I pray that the person reading this book will also crave order and maintenance. I pray that, if they enter into the profession of nursing, they will honor You by continuously seeking truth and maintaining order as they serve Your children.

In Jesus' Holy and most precious name, Amen.

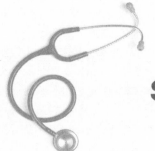

Chapter 16

Sights, Sounds, Smells . . . Oh My!

H ave you ever walked by someone wearing a certain perfume or cologne and were instantly taken back to a moment in time? Or maybe the smell of fresh-baked banana bread holds such a distinct memory that you can actually close your eyes and visualize your mama bending over in front of the stove with her oven mitts, and your five-year-old self salivating profusely, eagerly awaiting the first bite. The sound of fried chicken sizzling in a pan of grease, the exhaust fan roaring above the stove, and Monday night wrestling buzzing on the TV in the background instantaneously take me back to my childhood nights sleeping over with all of my cousins at my grandparents' house. Jesus spoke of remembrance to the disciples at the Lord's Supper. He told them that the "cup is the new covenant in my blood. Do this . . . in remembrance of me" (1 Corinthians 11:25). That is why, in many churches, people take the Lord's Supper, breaking bread and drinking wine or grape juice. It is done as a reminder of Jesus' death on the Cross, His Resurrection, and the promise of His return.

The brain is an intricately detailed, strategically designed organ. It is fascinating to me that the human mind possesses the ability to retrieve such vivid memories based on simplistic sensory stimuli. The brain not only has the capability to retrieve information based on sensory stimulation, but it also has the ability to desensitize your nose to lingering smells, your ears to monotonous noises, and your eyes to certain levels of lighting. This stimulated information retrieval or desensitizing disappearance of sights, sounds, or smells may be welcomed or unwelcomed.

For instance, have you ever gone over to a friend's house and the smell of their wet dog smacked you in the face the moment you entered the front door? However, once you were there for an hour or so, the smell seemed to disappear, despite the fact that the dog was lying right under your feet? This was probably a welcomed desensitization. Thank you, way to go, brain! This type of sensory desensitization can also be celebrated in nursing. For example, when a nurse is caring for a patient with uncontrollable diarrhea, we welcome the desensitization of our noses to the not-so-pleasant smell. Nonetheless, there are those people who are gifted, or perhaps cursed, with the sense of smell similar to that of a German shepherd. In these instances, a little essential oil of lavender or peppermint dabbed under each nostril helps tremendously.

The sense of smell is not the only sense where nurses can experience desensitization. After hours and hours of phones ringing, call lights dinging, and monitors beeping, a nurse's sense of hearing also seems to diminish. We can develop what many refer to as alarm fatigue. This is where a nurse has heard a sound for so long that the brain somehow begins to block the stimuli, and the sounds are no longer noticed. This can be extremely dangerous! Picture this. A nurse is caring for a patient on a cardiac monitor and their alarm has been sounding all evening for minor, non-life-threatening cardiac rates. It has not been necessary for the nurse to intervene. However, all of a sudden the patient enters into a life-threatening rhythm. The nurse is already experiencing alarm fatigue and fails to react to the alarm. The patient could die and the nurse would be responsible. That is why it is vital for nurses to take periodic mental breaks to refresh themselves. This can be as simple as walking into the restroom, closing your eyes, and taking ten deep breaths in the silence. Just this short mental break can be enough to rejuvenate the mind and lessen the effects of alarm fatigue.

Nurses need enhanced auditory sensation as well as perceptive visual recognition. As mentioned in chapter 3, some people have various sights that produce anxiety or a negative physiological response. However, similar to smells, certain sights can be clues as to what is going on within a patient's body. Thus, nurses must remain aware at all times. For example, if a child develops a rash on their torso with an elevated temperature and an inability to swallow food, a prudent nurse that has visualized this in previous encounters might quickly recognize the rash as the "scarlet fever rash" related to strep throat, and implement the appropriate interventions. However, a nurse who has never before been exposed to this type of rash or lacks the remembrance factor might miss the diagnosis all together. Hence, this is why Jesus said to the disciples as often as they drink the cup and break the bread that they do so in "remembrance" of Him. Memories are connected to emotion and sensory stimulation.

It is quite obvious why a nurse requires a keen sense of vision and hearing, coupled with the ability to remember and connect. We have to observe objective information with our eyes and listen intently to subjective information with our ears in order to make accurate assessments and develop appropriate interventions. However, you may be questioning the rationale supporting the requirement of a nurse's astute sense of smell. Although many smells are unpleasant in the profession of nursing, several medical conditions can actually be identified through smell. Once a nurse has caught his or her first waft of a gastrointestinal bleed, diarrhea resulting from Clostridium difficile (a highly contagious infection), or a wound infected with pseudomonas (a bacteria), he or she will never forget it. It is similar to the memory attached to the cologne or banana bread mentioned at the beginning of this chapter, but not quite so pleasurable. In countless instances, it is a nurse's sense of smell that leads to the recognition of these ailments, so that they may be reported to the primary healthcare provider for treatment plan development.

The importance of utilizing these sensory encounters (sights, sounds, and smells) as clues to aid in problem recognition is crucial. Nurses must nurture their senses, initiating visual, auditory, and olfactory breaks to avoid missing important clues when assessing patients. However, nurses must also avoid feeling guilty when cologne and banana bread are not exactly the smells wafting down the hospital hallway, and a little lavender oil under the nose is mandatory to make it through the shift.

My Prayer for You

Heavenly Father,

Thank You so much for creating us with such intricately detailed, strategically designed brains. Thank You for the sense of smell, sight, and hearing. What incredible assets to possess in the profession of nursing! I pray that, each time I am caring for a patient I will utilize all of my senses in order to determine the best care necessary. As the person reading this book encounters sensory stimuli that recalls various memories, I pray that they are pleasant memories or memories that will help them in their journey of helping others through nursing. May we remember You often and do everything as if unto You, always.

In Jesus' Holy and most precious name, Amen.

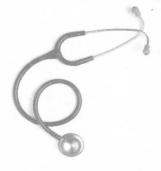

Chapter 17

Death and Dying: A Heavy Heart

Humans are finite beings. Despite the thought processes of many, we are not supernatural nor invincible. When I started this book several months ago, I still believed in my heart and mind that my earthly daddy was indestructible. He was a mountain of a man, six feet five inches tall and over 350 pounds. His hands were huge! Society is impressed with basketball players who can palm a basketball. Well, my daddy could palm a car battery, which can weigh 40 pounds or more. Some people equated him to a giant redwood tree. He was a strong man whose outer bark seemed rough, but in the center he was all sap. I knew the key to my daddy's heart and was well-acquainted with his soft side.

Although he was soft on the inside, my daddy was a hard-working man. He owned his own car salvage business, and I cannot remember a day that he was not under the hood of a car or behind the wheel of a wrecker or car hauler. His hands were as tough as leather, scarred from the years of manual labor, and seldom was there not some amount of grease under his nails. Working with my daddy was often the highlight of my week. At the age of four, my first job at the salvage was to pick up nuts and bolts off of the ground and place them in five gallon buckets. As I grew older, I graduated to new jobs, eventually running the entire business when daddy had to go out of town. I was daddy's "little grease monkey" as he liked to refer to me.

Daddy's little grease monkey was the greatest title I ever earned. Pulling car parts and getting covered in the black sticky grease that was often caked under old car hoods brought me great joy. Daddy was so proud that I was passionate about his

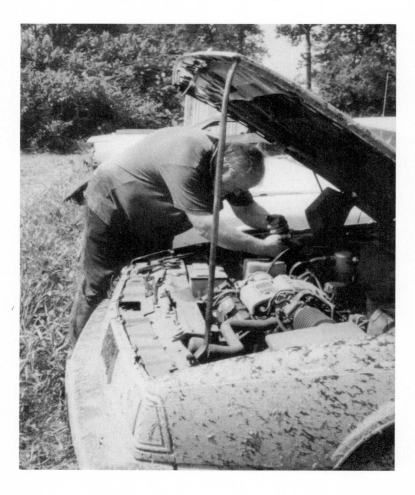

passion. I loved my daddy so much that I would have done anything to make him proud. My daddy taught me everything about cars. He taught me the key elements to running a successful business. He taught me how to work hard and how to play hard. My daddy taught me more than this book has pages to hold. As I said before, in my heart, my daddy was going to live forever because the thought of living without him seemed nearly impossible.

However, "All flesh is like grass and all its glory like the flower of the grass. The grass withers, and the flower falls" (1 Peter 1:24). After only 58 years of life, my daddy's body withered and his flesh failed him. For years, my daddy suffered from high blood pressure and diabetes, which eventually caused his kidneys to stop working and led to blindness in the right eye and near blindness in the left eye. In chapter 4, I discussed the disappearance of my daddy's sight. At the time I wrote that chapter, he was still functioning in society. He walked with a cane, but was still able to go places and enjoy life. Little did I know that, by the time I reached chapter 17, my daddy would be gone from this earth forever. Genesis 3:19 says that "By the sweat of your face you shall eat bread, till you return to the ground, for out of it you were taken; for you are dust, and to dust you shall return."

The last several months of my daddy's life included a gradual loss of independence and degradation of dignity. He became completely dependent on others to take him places, assist him to and from vehicles, and even to dial his phone. The big, hard-working, independent, business-owning, strong, indestructible mountain of a man was now reliant on everyone but himself. I could visibly see and almost tangibly feel the pain and sorrow that plagued him. He grew bitter about living. Dialysis three times per week for five hours each day was not exactly how he had envisioned life at 58, but it was, in fact, his reality. I recall my daddy stating on many occasions, "I'm either going to have to get busy living or get busy dying. I can't do this in-between stuff anymore."

The daughter in me wanted him to get busy living. The nurse in me desperately desired to "fix" everything so that dying was not an option. I would clean my daddy's apartment, wash his dishes, do his laundry, complete dressing changes on his diabetic foot ulcerations, and assist him with bathing around the tubes and lines connected to his body for dialysis treatments. Anything that would make his life seemingly easier, I was willing to do it. After my many lectures about how negatively certain foods would affect his blood sugar, we would, all too often, at daddy's request, chow down on cheeseburgers and ice cream for supper. That was what brought him joy in the last weeks and months of his life.

In fact, September 26, 2014, the evening of my 32nd birthday, I prepared my daddy a bologna sandwich, sliced bell peppers and tomatoes, an apple, and a glass of milk. I handed him his sandwich, placed his other food, as well as his phone, on the table next to him, explaining where each thing was located so that he was able to feel it since his vision was so poor. It seemed weird when he said that he could see everything and that I just needed to leave, but nonetheless, I rubbed his shoulder and said, "I love you, Daddy," as I walked out of his apartment completely unaware that those moments were the last ones that I would ever experience with my daddy this side of heaven.

My plan was to only be gone for a little while and return to administer his evening medications and ensure that he was okay for the night. However, as I sat in a restaurant eating my birthday supper with my husband, a startling, paralyzing fear came over my body. "Suddenly, I feel like something is very wrong with my daddy. We need to leave right away," I whispered to my husband as I choked back tears. Then, literally seconds after that statement, my husband's cell phone rang. It was my mama. She said we needed to come quick. My daddy was unconscious and the paramedics were working diligently to revive him.

His neighbors had done as I instructed. They had checked on him every 20 to 30 minutes. One gentleman had brought him chicken and ice cream only an hour or so after I had left him. When the neighbor found my daddy's lifeless body face down in the kitchen, there was the carton of ice cream with the spoon still in it next to his chair. This is the way he would have wanted it. His last supper was ice cream.

As I pulled into daddy's apartment complex, I was quickly reminded that only God can breathe life into a human being and by His grace alone would my daddy breathe again. However, that was not His plan on that September night. His plan was to allow my daddy to leave his tired, worn-out shell of a body behind and be joined with Him in heaven. He is probably eating the richest, creamiest, most flavorful ice cream ever now!

As nurses, we must pay attention to what is important in end-of-life care. We must remember that the human lying in the bed we are looming over might be a daddy, a son, a mother, or a daughter. That person once had a career and grandiose dreams for life. They probably were known by their family as strong and invincible. I am in no way expressing that we jeopardize someone's life for a bowl of ice cream. However, if they are in the end stages of a disease process and they find their joy in a bowl of ice cream, it is at that point we must make a decision as to what is morally right: strict maintenance of a bland, low sodium, low sugar diet or allowance of a one-time moment of indulgence.

As discussed in an earlier chapter, there are a multitude of various levels and types of nursing careers. However, caring for someone at the end of life is one of the greatest honors and privileges that could ever be bestowed upon a human being. Although I was not actually my daddy's nurse, I have had the privilege of being the nurse of many people near the end of their earthly lives. Nursing care at the end of life is often referred to as palliative care. To palliate is to offer oneself and services in order to make the effects of something less painful, harmful, or harsh.[1]

Hospice nurses specialize in palliative care. They visit patients' homes, nursing care facilities, and hospitals to ensure that the dying person receives the most appropriate, effective, palliative care. This may include pain medications to alleviate intractable pain. It may be music therapy, soft lighting, and specialty beds or pillows to increase comfort. It may be offering prayer or contacting the patient's religious leader. It may be feeding them a bowl of ice cream!

Caring for someone at the end of life is not an easy task. It takes selflessness. It takes compassion. It takes love! Humans are complex. We are not invincible! However, we are physical, emotional, and spiritual beings that require nurturing, especially when we are no longer able to nurture ourselves.

My Prayer for You

Heavenly Father,

First of all, I want to praise You for the 32 years that You allowed me to have with my earthly father. Thank You for a daddy who loved me unconditionally and taught me so much. I know that my daddy is gone from this earth, but I am thankful that Your Holy Spirit remains with me to comfort and provide me with peace that passes all understanding. I pray that the person reading this book knows and willingly accepts the same peace and comfort. Perhaps they never

1. Merriam- Webster Online Dictionary, http://www.merriam-webster.com/.

knew their earthly father, or maybe they are still enjoying wonderful moments with him, or just maybe they
are caring for their dying daddy right now. No matter
their circumstance, I pray that they feel Your presence
and are intimately acquainted with Your perfect peace.
Father, if the person reading this book dedicates their
life to nursing, I pray that they will strive to make every
moment count, especially when privileged with caring
for Your children as they are transitioning from this life
into eternity.

In Jesus' Holy and most precious name, Amen.

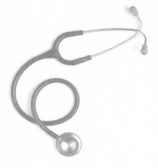

Chapter 18

Mind, Body, Spirit: Triune Care

Awise gentleman recently spoke to the students in my sophomore Holistic Assessment nursing course. I invite him to speak to my class each year in order to help the students better comprehend how to obtain a thorough spiritual patient assessment. This extraordinary gentleman has a doctorate in divinity and worked as a church pastor and college chaplain for many years. However, he is currently a full-time assistant professor of Biblical and Theological Studies. Therefore, he is highly qualified to fulfill the endeavor of teaching spiritual assessment.

This year, he confidently walked into my class with a hot cup of earl gray tea in his hand. His suit was crisp and freshly laundered complete with a tie. With silver hair and the college insignia embroidered on the left breast of his suit jacket, he appeared distinguished and wise. After I introduced him to the class, the man immediately said in a soft, yet certain tone of voice, "There are two kinds of nurses: those who enter their patients' rooms and simply do their jobs like a checklist, and those who actually care." He walked throughout the classroom, weaving in and out of desks, making eye contact with each student. This captured the students' attention rather quickly. I noticed that they were hanging on every word and eagerly anticipating where this presentation was going to go next.

The man continued by instructing the students to pretend that they had already graduated from the nursing program, had successfully passed the NCLEX-RN exam, and were assigned to care for a patient in the ICU named "Pat." He explained Pat's situation in great detail. She had checked into the hospital believing that the signs and symptoms plaguing her body were merely manifestations of the flu. However, once admitted, the healthcare professionals quickly discovered that Pat did not have the flu, but was actually experiencing kidney, as well as multiple other body system failures. Additionally, the one attempt at hemodialysis (a procedure that cleanses the blood through a machine similar to how a kidney functions) had induced Pat's second stroke in her five-day hospitalization.

The gentleman continued sharing Pat's story, explaining how many nurses entered and exited her hospital room, paying little attention to much more than her physical condition. They were just there to do a job, collect a paycheck, and go home. It was obvious that he was choking back tears when his voice broke as he spoke of how no one noticed that Pat had not received flowers, balloons, or other typical "get well" gifts. Furthermore, although it was Pat lying ill in the hospital bed, the one and only, single, solitary card that was gently propped open in the windowsill was addressed to Pat's husband and not Pat. The man explained that Pat appeared increasingly frustrated, agitated, and even fearful at times.

Pat's eyes darted wildly as she examined every individual who walked into her room. She struggled to speak, and when she did, no one was there to listen. She was trapped in her failing body and there was nothing that she could do to stop the decline. Not one nurse had taken the time to ask Pat about her fears or attempted to address any concerns that she may have possessed. No one from a church had visited, and the hospital chaplain had not been notified. Pat's daughter had driven several hours to be at her mother's bedside. However, her face was plagued with emotion demonstrative of distant, hurtful memories. Nonetheless, she stared lovingly into her mother's face. She realized that all of the years of self-medication were not to cure Pat's physical pain, but more to blunt the emotional and spiritual agony that haunted her for so long.

The man slowly walked about the classroom sipping his hot earl gray tea as he made eye contact again with each and every nursing student. It was obvious that he had their attention. He certainly had mine. I was enamored with his story and somewhat infuriated that none of the nurses had taken the time to address the obvious internal emotional and spiritual battle that Pat had been fighting for years and was continuing to fight as she lie there nearing what could be the end of her life. My mind wondered, where was Pat going to spend eternity? Did no one care that she might die with unfinished business, unanswered questions, and unresolved anger? Did no one realize that "the body apart from the spirit is dead" (James 2:26)? Were the nurses blind, deaf, and mute?! I doubt the nurses were physically blind, deaf, or mute. However, they were obviously oblivious to the nonverbal cues that Pat was emanating.

The gentleman speaker leaned against a desk positioned at the front of the classroom. His lips parted slightly and formed a reminiscent smile. I could tell that the pivotal moment in Pat's story was about to occur. The students shifted uncomfortably in their chairs as if preparing for the climax of an intense action-packed Hollywood movie. I did not realize it, but I had scooted myself to the edge of my seat as well. We all breathed a sigh of relief as the man spoke the words, "No one had taken the time to assess and uncover the meaning behind the years of Pat's self-medication, the rationale behind her lack of visitors, the reason why her one card was addressed to her husband, or why her daughter's face was plagued with torment, until that one nurse who actually cared entered Pat's room."

He went on to explain how that special nurse took the time to sit down next to the hospital bed, gently grasp Pat's hand, and ask her the questions she so desperately longed to answer. Although Pat struggled to speak, she was responsive to the nurse's words and touch. The nurse never really had to speak of Jesus. She simply loved Pat as she imagined He would love Pat. She demonstrated care and concern, not only for Pat's mind and body, but also for her spirit.

> But if Christ is in you, although the body is dead because of sin, the Spirit is life because of righteousness. If the Spirit of him who raised Jesus from the dead dwells in you, he who raised Christ Jesus from the dead will also give life to your mortal bodies through his Spirit who dwells in you (Romans 8:10–11).

Although the nurse assisted Pat in the physical dying process as she cleansed her face, emptied her drainage bags, and administered her medications, she was really offering her life, assisting her with finding closure, giving her the freedom to die. Without a physical body, Pat would have never been able to live and breathe here on earth. Without a mind, she would not have been able to think or function in society. Without a soul, she would have never had the capacity to love, the ability to know happiness or joy, and ultimately, the capability to experience reconciliation with her family.

As the gentleman addressing my class brought Pat's story to a close, he revealed that Pat was his mother-in-law, that the daughter with years of unresolved anguish from hurt inflicted by Pat's bitterness was his wife, and that the one nurse who took the time to pay attention to Pat's body, mind, and spirit was an angel in his family's mind. Tears ran down his cheeks as he expressed his and his family's gratitude for the nurse who paid attention to the triune aspect of life: mind, body, spirit. He explained that Pat died shortly after the caring nurse spoke with her and assisted her in the resolution of much of her painful past. Furthermore, he expressed to the students that his family sent the nurse a check thanking her for going above and beyond the call of duty.

As the class full of future nurses sat silently soaking in the story of Pat's life and death, I pondered: did that "special" nurse really do anything "special"? Were her actions miraculous? My response was "no." That nurse had done what was right. She recognized that the body cannot truly live without the mind and the spirit, but the body also cannot die when the mind and spirit are in a state of unrest.

The distinguished, doctorally prepared, wise gentleman presented the story of Pat in a way that personalized it for the students. I am sure that they will not quickly forget about Pat, if ever. He walked into a classroom full of young men and women who may have believed that nursing was just the physical act of providing patient care, but he walked out of a classroom full of people acutely aware of how much holistic triune care truly matters.

My Prayer for You

Heavenly Father,

Thank You so much for being a Triune God: God the Father, God the Son (Jesus), and God the Holy Spirit. Thank You for Ms. Pat and her story. Thank You for a nurse who cared and took the time to address all three aspects of the human: mind, body, spirit. I pray that the students sitting in my class that day will become nurses who pay attention to all aspects of their patients' care, who will serve their patients' minds, bodies, and spirits. I also ask these things for the person reading this book. Father, give them a heart for people. Help them see beyond the bitterness and the pain expressed by their patients. Give them the ability to provide genuine holistic, triune care in a world that often views healthcare as the restoration of physical bodily function. Let them cause a ripple effect throughout the nursing profession just as a smooth stone thrown into a pond creates beautiful ripples that permeate all the way to the shore.

In Jesus' Holy and most precious name, Amen.

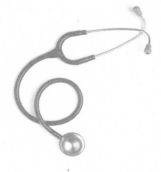

Chapter 19

Creating a Nourishing Environment

The hair on the back of Kylie's neck stood straight up. She gritted her teeth and clenched her fists, as she slowly and sharply inhaled. She was making a valiant attempt to calm herself from the frustration and discouragement she was experiencing in that moment. Kylie had worked in the same nursing home for 22 years, but two weeks ago she accepted the position of administrator and was quickly finding out that not everyone internalized the same beliefs, values, and ideals that she did. For 22 years, Kylie had done her job as if unto the Lord. She came in early, stayed late, and loved each resident as if they were her own family member. However, when she was working as a nurse, she was unaware of the actions of many of the other staff members.

Now, as the administrator, she was becoming acutely aware that the environment of the nursing home was quite uncomfortable and downright hostile at times. The walls were gray, the floors dingy, the smells horrific, and the staff seemed to only come to work for the weekly paycheck. Their expressions were smug, their shoulders slumped downward, and their words like two-edged swords. Often, the hurtful words of the staff were directed toward the residents and one another.

Kylie remained quiet for the first couple of weeks as administrator. She wanted to carefully observe and gather information before she devised a plan. She was cognizant of the monumental job that lay before her, but did not want to institute any drastic changes prematurely and without wisdom. She knew that "wisdom is better than jewels, and all that you may desire cannot compare with her" (Proverbs 8:11).

During the two-week observation period, Kylie noticed many things. She carried around a small notepad and ink pen everywhere she went, taking diligent notes. She noticed the staff looked tired and worn out. They had bags under their eyes, and their uniforms were often wrinkled and unkempt. Some uniforms did not even match or were noticeably too small. She also noticed that many of the nursing assistants were working 16-hour shifts and unable to take a complete lunch break due to staffing issues. Kylie was astonished when she visited with several staff members that did not even know each other's names. She thought to herself, "This is unacceptable." With her pen in hand, she jotted down — "Create plan to encourage staff bonding," then carried on gingerly, observing every detail of the physical, emotional, and spiritual environment throughout the nursing home.

Kylie pondered what could have possibly gone so wrong that the staff, who had worked together for years, did not even care enough to learn about their colleagues. If they did not know their colleagues' names, what did they not know about the residents? She thought about it for a moment. Over the last several years, the administrative staff had aged and lacked the zeal they once had regarding the care of the residents. They had turned deaf ears and blind eyes when the building needed attention, the staff would cut corners, and residents' families would complain. However, Kylie whispered to herself quietly, "Things are about to change around here." And by change, she meant for the better.

As Kylie went back to her office and closed the door, she looked around the room. She had beautiful pictures of family, friends, and oceanic scenery covering the walls. A candle flickered on her desk that wafted a beautiful aroma into the air. Before she had moved into the office, she had the walls covered with a fresh coat of soft blue paint. The blue made her think of the sky on a clear, sunny day. And the lamp on the corner of her desk offered alternate soft, comforting lighting in lieu of the harsh fluorescent lights overhead.

No wonder she loved her office! It was warm, inviting, comfortable, and nourishing. A smile crossed her face as new ideas for the nursing home flooded her mind. Invigoration and deep compassion filled her heart as she was reminded, "Whatever you wish that others would do to you, do also to them" (Matthew 7:12). No one has the ability to nourish others without first being nourished themselves. She would start by nourishing the staff, so that, in turn, they could nourish the residents living in the facility.

Kylie leapt to her feet, humming to the tune that was playing on her office computer as she bounced back out into the hallway to start creating a nourishing environment for the people she was now responsible for. If "the Son of Man came not to be served but to serve, and to give his life as a ransom for many" (Matthew 20:28), she could serve the people of the nursing home which God had placed in her authority.

The first thing she did was clean out one of the old storage rooms, paint the walls with some of the paint left over from her office, and strategically place soft comfy chairs and couches around the room. The couches and chairs had been donated by one of the resident's family years ago, but had remained piled up in storage. They were about to be put to good use. Kylie brought in a lamp and area rug from home, and placed soothing pictures of the ocean and mountains on each of the walls. Three days later, she slowly examined every inch of the new employee lounge and smiled with great pleasure. This new "sacred space" would hopefully provide a place to nourish the hearts and souls of the staff and offer a room where they could go to relax, debrief, pray, and reflect.

Kylie's next order of business was to join the staff together more closely. This was going to be a difficult chore, but one for which she was ready. She created posters advertising an "appreciation party" for the staff. The posters delineated that each shift would have their own parties in the *"Newly Created Sacred Space Lounge."* Kylie had gotten the administrative staff and volunteers to cover the care of the residents while the parties transpired. After all, the staff needed to know that they were valued and it was time for upper management to serve the frontline staff.

As the glorious day approached, Kylie's excitement and enthusiasm increased. She had worked diligently to be present every day, answering questions, being responsive, and showing kindness and compassion to the staff. She prayed that they had noticed her efforts in trying to listen to their requests and nourish their souls. Kylie took some money from the master operating budget and had a variety of beautiful, aromatic foods catered and delivered on the day of the big event. She had surveyed the staff regarding their favorite foods and had ordered them accordingly. Kylie had also ordered each staff member two new uniforms with their names and credentials embroidered over their hearts. She personally wrapped each one in bright yellow paper and placed an orange bow on top. She wanted the gifts to represent a new beginning, like the sunshine on the dawn of a new day. It was Kylie's hope that these gestures would encourage and inspire the staff.

The day of the scheduled parties, the staff buzzed around like bees in a hive. They were not exactly sure what to expect. Some thought the "appreciation party" was symbolic of a "farewell party." They thought that there were about to be more staff and budget cuts. Others thought it was a meeting to reprimand them, disguised as a party. Others just weren't sure what to expect. However, one by one, as they entered the Sacred Space Lounge, eyes grew big like saucers, mouths fell open in disbelief, and many were speechless. The smell of wonderful foods permeated the room. Soft, soothing music filled the air. Brightly colored gifts covered a large table in the corner. And there stood Kylie, their boss, with a huge smile planted across her face. "Welcome, come on in and get comfortable," she said to each one as they entered.

Shift by shift, it was the same response. The staff members entered with astonishment written all over their faces. After their bellies were full of great food, they had opened their new uniforms, and they appeared to have an expression of satisfaction, Kylie spoke with confidence, kindness, and compassion. She explained her heart and the desire she had to create a nourishing environment for them, so that, in turn, they could create a nourishing environment for the residents and each other.

She further explained that more staff members would soon be hired to decrease the workload of individuals; upgrades would be made throughout the building; new equipment would be purchased to make their jobs easier; and laundry services would be offered to launder their uniforms. She also expressed to each staff member the value that they held and how they made a difference in the lives of the residents and other staff members. She announced that there would be monthly staff meetings that included a built-in time for fellowship to encourage them to get to know each other on a deeper, more intimate level. Kylie's hope was that these times of fellowship would knit the staff more closely together and encourage teamwork. She also pointed out that her office had an "open door" policy and that she was always available to discuss any comments or concerns. Furthermore, she placed a secured box in the Sacred Space Lounge for anonymous comments. Kylie explained that she would personally collect these comments on a weekly basis and that each comment would undergo careful consideration.

The staff expressed how pleased they were with the new changes and attention to their concerns. The air seemed lighter. Everyone was buzzing around smiling, laughing, and visiting. This is exactly what Kylie had anticipated. As the weeks went by, Kylie continued to maintain the nourishing environment of the nursing home and hold true to her promises. Many upgrades were made. New resident lifts, blood pressure cuffs, and medication administration carts were purchased and being utilized. The staff members were working as a team, helping each other and not going against the grain. Several of the residents even expressed their satisfaction with the increasingly pleasant environment and staff demeanor.

As Kylie sat in her office, she reflected on the recent improvements. She had known that a person's environment could affect their attitude and actions, but she just had not realized how drastically. By paying attention to detail, listening to others' thoughts, recognizing the need for change, and making a goal to create a nourishing environment, Kylie had demonstrated respect, placed high value on the staff, restored teamwork, and, ultimately, revolutionized the care provided to the residents. This brought her great joy. She smiled and breathed in a deep sigh of relief as she thanked God for His example and petitioned Him to continuously nourish her soul, so that she could, in turn, nourish others.

My Prayer for You

Heavenly Father,

It is Your desire to comfort and nourish us through the presence of the Holy Spirit. Without the Holy Spirit dwelling within us, and remaining in constant communion and communication with You, we are unable to remain filled, fulfilled, and nourished. If we are emotionally and spiritually starving, we have nothing to give to others. I pray that both the reader of this book and I will continuously seek You. I pray that we will know what is good, right, and true, and choose to always love one another as You love us. Help us to remain emotionally and spiritually nourished, so that we might be fully equipped to nourish those in our care.

In Jesus' Holy and most precious name, Amen.

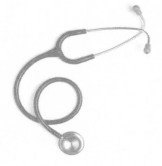

Chapter 20

Patients Require Patience

"HURRY UP! YOU PEOPLE ARE RIDICULOUS! YOU DON'T EVEN KNOW WHAT YOU ARE DOING! I HATE THIS PLACE!" my patient screamed, along with various other obscenities, as he was being wheeled on the stretcher down the long corridor to the hospital room to which he had been assigned. I swallowed hard, took a deep breath, and sighed heavily as I thought to myself sarcastically, "Just great! This is going to be a long night." It was my turn for the next admission, and I guess I drew the short straw that night. The yelling, screaming, belligerent man was my new patient.

I had cared for many patients throughout my career, patients of all shapes and sizes with varying personalities and preferences, but none quite like this man. As I sat at the nurses' station reviewing the patient's new admission orders, labs, and radiology reports, I could still hear him bellowing down the hallway, griping with every breath. Once the transport personnel and nursing assistants had gotten him settled, I walked hesitantly down the hall into my patient's room.

As I peered through the doorway, there he sat in bed, a scowling grimace covering his face. I examined him carefully as I approached his bedside. He was a giant, burly man with a long gray beard and gray, thinning hair. He appeared much older than his young 63 years. I assumed this was related to a hard-lived life. His body was as round as Santa Claus, but his belly was not jiggling like a bowl full of jelly from laughter. No. He was a far cry from happy. My eyes scanned from the head all the way down to the foot of the bed. Nurses must examine every inch of a patient, especially when they are first admitted, as not to miss a single detail that could assist in providing excellent care.

When my eyes reached the man's legs, I noticed that he only had one leg, his left one. The right one had been amputated above the knee. I panned the room quickly to discover that his prosthesis lay on the chair beside him. My mind wondered momentarily what kind of life had this man endured, why was he so angry, what happened to his leg, and why was he living in a nursing home at only 63 years old? Little did I know, these questions would soon be answered, if I only had the patience to wait for the hard shell that was covering his heart to melt away. Just as I was telling myself that I could do that because the Lord has commanded that we "love one another," and that "love is patient and kind" (John 13:34; 1 Corinthians 13:4), my thoughts came to a screeching halt when the patient yelled at me, "WHO ARE YOU AND WHAT EXACTLY ARE YOU DOING HERE?"

Startled, I breathed in sharply. "My name is Chelsia. I am going to be your nurse for the remainder of the evening until 7:00 in the morning," I said in the sweetest tone I could possibly muster at that point. After all, "A soft answer turns away wrath, but a harsh word stirs up anger" (Proverbs 15:1). I confidently stuck my right hand out to shake his. He seemed shocked, but obliged and shook my hand. I explained that I was the nurse assigned to care for him throughout the night and assured him that I was there to take care of him in the best possible way. I further explained that "his wish was my command." He needed to have a sense of control and I was going to provide that for him.

Hour after hour went by, and each time I would walk into the patient's room, he would make rude, disrespectful remarks, or simply ignore me when I tried to engage in conversation with him. However, each time, I approached him from a position of love and respect. If he made a rude comment, I would respond to him with a kind tone and demeanor. Although I wanted to avoid him like the plague, something inside of me yearned to know more about him. I wanted to help him.

At 2:00 a.m., after all of my patients' evening medications were administered, their pillows were fluffed, and they were tucked in and resting quietly, I decided to peek in on the angry old man. There he was, wide eyed, staring at the television. I glanced up to see what he was watching. I was shocked to see that it was a late-night evangelist preaching the gospel of Jesus Christ. What an oxymoron, I thought. This mean, hateful, rude, disrespectful man was watching a gospel message. I slowly and carefully walked into his room and began assessing his oxygen tubing connection and picking up some trash that he had thrown onto the floor. Just as I bent over to pick up the last piece of trash, I heard a quiet, broken voice say, "Ma'am, can I talk to you?" It couldn't be. Surely, I was just hearing things. The man in that bed had an angry, loud, boisterous voice. That kind, quiet voice could not have just come from him.

As I rose up slowly, I caught a glimpse of the man's face. His cheeks were tear-stained and tears were still actively flowing down from his eyes. My heart ached for him. "Yes sir. I am here for you. What would you like to talk about?" I questioned.

In that moment, every ounce of anger, fear, and frustration left his face. He was broken. Through sobs, he asked for my forgiveness, acknowledging his disrespectfulness toward me. "I have been so hateful to you all night and you have just been trying to do your job. You have been patient with and kind to me. I'm sorry for the way that I have acted," he spoke softly. If I could have leapt for joy in that moment, I would have, but that might not have been very professional. So, I just placed my hand over his, smiled warmly, and said, "Don't you worry. I forgive you. You just do not feel well. When someone does not feel well, they act in ways that are atypical."

He returned my smile with a half-hearted grin. "Thank you," he said, "but, you did not deserve to be treated the way I have treated you. I am a Christian and should never have acted the way I did toward you."

Before I realized it, we had been lost in conversation for almost an hour and an half. This hurting, broken man had shared his heartaches with me regarding the loss of his fiancé in a tragic car accident months before he had his leg amputated, and how that trial had been the road to his declining health and admission into a nursing home. His anger and bitterness ran deep. He had much resentment toward God and other people. He did not understand why he had endured such tragedy and others seemed to be enjoying abundant blessings.

I made a desperate attempt to comfort him, sharing some of the tragedies that I had endured throughout life and how I had coped. He seemed to cling to every word I spoke, as if it were the next doorway to his happiness. I knew that I could not give him false hope, but that I could give him some hope; the hope that God was still with him and that often through illness, heartache, and tribulations our faith becomes solidified. James 1:2–3 says, "Count it all joy, my brothers, when you meet trials of various kinds, for you know that the testing of your faith produces steadfastness."

The trial of caring for a cantankerous old man that night certainly produced steadfastness of my own faith. As I sat down next to him, held his hands in mine, and obeyed the command from God to "confess your sins to one another and pray for one another" (James 5:16), my heart was forever changed. In the very room, from the same lips that had cursed me earlier, I heard, not the boisterous, hateful voice, but the trembling, soft voice of a man whose faith was being restored, pray for me.

That loud, demanding, hateful patient required much patience that night. (And there have been many more since him.) However, all the time, energy, and perseverance paid off. Each time he was admitted to the hospital, he would bellow all the way down the hallways, "IF CHELSIA CAN'T BE MY NURSE, I'M NOT STAYING!" The other nurses gladly obliged his requests, and often looked at me with bewilderment when a genuine smile came across my face every time I saw his name pop up on the patient census.

As I have said several times throughout this book, nursing is more than a profession. It is more than a job. It is even more than a career. Nursing is a calling. We deal with imperfect human beings who are often hurting, sick, sad, and downright angry. We must daily remind ourselves that nurses require *patients* in order to earn a living, but we require *patience* in order to fulfill our calling.

My Prayer for You

> Heavenly Father,
> Thank You for setting an example of patience. As human beings, we fail You each day, but Your mercy endures forever. You are so gracious and forgiving. Please forgive me when my patience has worn thin and

I was too quick to respond in anger. Help me to continually grow in patience as I serve Your children. Father, if the person reading this book devotes their life to the calling of nursing, I ask that You would also grant them the ability to remain patient, even with the most difficult of patients. After all, "Love is patient and kind; love does not envy or boast; it is not arrogant or rude. It does not insist on its own way; it is not irritable or resentful; it does not rejoice at wrongdoing, but rejoices with the truth. Love bears all things, believes all things, hopes all things, endures all things. Love never ends" (1 Corinthians 13:4–8).

In Jesus' Holy and most precious name, Amen.

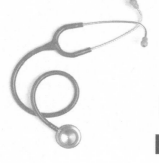

Chapter 21

Fatigued, but Not Finished: A Prescription for Perseverance

Jesus spent 33 years loving, serving, and offering compassion to others, many of whom were rude, disrespectful, or denied and even despised Him. He educated the uneducated, ministered to the lost and hurting, fed the hungry, gave sight to the blind, healed the sick, and even raised the dead. And, if that was not exhausting enough, Jesus knew His purpose and lived a sinless life, blameless before God, the Father.

On the day of Jesus' crucifixion, He endured pain and suffering far beyond anything we could ever imagine. He was brutally beaten beyond recognition. He was cursed at and spat on. He was stripped of His clothes, placed in a purple robe with a crown of thorns buried into His head as a form of royal mockery. The physical, emotional, and spiritual fatigue Jesus must have felt at that time is overwhelming to imagine. Yet, even as He was marching up the hill to Golgotha, where He was ultimately nailed to a Cross between two criminals, to be murdered, He continued to demonstrate unimaginable compassion saying, "Father, forgive them, for they know not what they do" (Luke 23:34).

We will never know, experience, or even be able to marginally comprehend the fatigue that Jesus felt on the day of His crucifixion. However, as human beings, we often experience physical, emotional, and spiritual fatigue and exhaustion. This is especially true among those working in the nursing profession. Nurses provide care to the sick and dying on a daily basis. As discussed in chapter 6, nurses can experience physical, emotional, and spiritual exhaustion. Physical exhaustion has the potential to decrease the quality of nursing care. However, when a nurse becomes so emotionally and spiritually exhausted that he or she no longer possesses the capacity to care, and are what many describe as "numb," nursing is no longer nursing.

This numbness, or inability to care, is often referred to as compassion fatigue. Compassion fatigue is the result of inveterate self-sacrifice. Nurses continuously provide care for sick, hurting, and even dying individuals. This repetition of exposure to trauma can induce or exacerbate compassion fatigue, leaving nurses unable to empathize with another's suffering and incapable of providing compassionate, nourishing care to patients.[1] The question is, how do we prevent or overcome this phenomenon?

Although there are many schools of thought, there are none that offer a concrete, black and white answer to this question. Since compassion fatigue is predominately an inward battle, it makes sense to combat it with internal weapons. I am not claiming to be an expert in the diagnosis, prevention, and treatment of compassion fatigue. However, I will say that, after 11 years in this profession, I can raise my right hand and honestly attest that I have not experienced compassion fatigue and do not currently possess compassion fatigue. Therefore, I will provide for

---

1. C. Harris and M.T. Quinn Griffin, "Nursing on Empty: Compassion Fatigue Signs, Symptoms, and System Interventions," *Journal of Christian Nursing*, 2015, 32(2), 2–9.

you the truth behind my personal resiliency to this potentially career-crippling ailment.

From the time that God called me to be a nurse until the present day, just as Jesus knew and fulfilled His purpose, I have known and continue to know that I have a purpose to fulfill here on this earth. First and foremost, I recognize and willingly accept the commandments to "Love the Lord [my] God with all [my] heart and with all [my] soul and with all [my] mind" and to "Love [my] neighbor as [myself]" (Matthew 22:37–39; NIV), keeping in mind that a neighbor is merely defined as a person who is *near* to another.[2] Since my patients are, obviously, *near* to me, they are considered my neighbors. Therefore, I am called to love them. But what does love look like? In the nursing profession, love can be manifested in many ways, but one of the most universal ways is through compassion. Compassionate nursing includes having a "sympathetic consciousness" of a patient's distress and possessing a deep desire to alleviate it.[3] Compassion is motivated by love. God is love. So, without God, our human nature is incapable of loving unconditionally, and thus, incapable of demonstrating honest, sincere compassion.

In order to demonstrate and offer constant, compassionate, unconditional love, I strive to be the nurse that I believe Jesus would be. This can be a struggle when dealing with "patients requiring patience." Therefore, I endeavor to nurture my relationship with God through devotional and Scripture reading, remaining in constant prayer and communion with the Lord, and listening intently to the Holy Spirit. I know it may sound cliché, but it truly is the only way that I can continue to give love. When a patience-requiring patient is demanding attention or being disrespectful, and I can feel my compassion for them dwindling, I stop, take a deep breath, and ask God to help me

---

2. Merriam- Webster Online Dictionary, http://www.merriam-webster.com/.
3. Ibid.

see the situation from their point of view. This automatically gives me a new, unjaded perspective, and refills my heart with love and compassion for them.

This is not only helpful with patients, but with all relationships. My marriage, relationships, and life are centered around and guided by the Holy Spirit within me. When Jesus was preparing the disciples for His departure, so that He could fulfill His purpose, He said to them, "If you love me, you will keep my commandments. And I will ask the Father, and he will give you another Helper, to be with you forever, even the Spirit of truth, whom the world cannot receive, because it neither sees him nor knows him. You know him, for he dwells with you and will be in you" (John 14:15–17). This Scripture is comforting and a constant reminder that I am not alone when faced with chronic patient trauma or death. The Holy Spirit is my personal internal motivator who assists me in combatting the spiritual battle of compassion fatigue.

Compassion fatigue inarguably is an inward spiritual battle. "For we do not wrestle against flesh and blood, but against the rulers, against the authorities, against the cosmic powers over this present darkness, against the spiritual forces of evil in the heavenly places" (Ephesians 6:12). You may be asking yourself, "How does one fight a spiritual battle?" Again, I am no expert, but I do know that striving to daily equip myself with internal weapons via the "armor of God" has protected me throughout my life and career.

> Therefore put on the full armor of God, so that when the day of evil comes, you may be able to stand your ground, and after you have done everything, to stand. Stand firm then, with the belt of truth buckled around your waist, with the breastplate of righteousness in place, and with your feet fitted with the readiness that comes from the gospel of peace. In addition

to all this, take up the shield of faith, with which you can extinguish all the flaming arrows of the evil one. Take the helmet of salvation and the sword of the spirit, which is the word of God. And pray in the Spirit on all occasions with all kinds of prayers and requests (Ephesians 6:13–18; NIV).

The Bible illustrates the invisible, animate qualities of truth, righteousness, peace, faith, salvation, and spirit in relationship to visible, inanimate objects. This vivid illustration helps to solidify the necessity of possessing and implementing these characteristics in life. First, to seek truth is to read, know, and understand Scripture. This is a process that takes daily, consistent reading and meditation. Once truth is fastened on tightly, like a belt, then righteousness follows. Righteousness includes remaining steadfast in regard to high moral standards. Humans are not innately righteous. The righteousness of God is manifested in us through our faith in Christ Jesus. A life of righteousness helps guard the heart, "for everything you do flows from it," like a breastplate (Proverbs 4:23; NIV).

A person with a peaceful heart leaves footprints of peace wherever they go. However, the evil one will try to rob people of their love and compassion for others, but faith in Jesus Christ and His living Word provides a shield deflecting the fatigue of such things. Although faith acts as protection for the heart, the mind can still fall victim to deceit. Thus, the gift of salvation, which is our rescue from the evil one, acts as a helmet of protection for the mind. Finally, the words of the Lord, scripted on the heart and inscribed in the mind, can act as a sword when faced with trauma and difficult situations threatening to fatigue someone of their compassion.

There is only one prescription for perseverance with regard to unconditional compassionate love — Jesus Christ. He was the ultimate portrayal of undefiled, pure, genuine, unconditional love. He knew His fate, to be murdered and die an unimaginable death on a Cross. However, He also knew His purpose, to save those who were (and are) lost and doomed for an eternity in hell. He loved us so much that He surrendered His life. Now, we must "remain in [His] love" so, that our "joy may be complete" (John 15:9–11; NIV). We fulfill this by obeying Jesus' command to love each other as He loved us because "Greater love has no one than this: to lay down one's life for one's friends" (John 15:12–13; NIV).

As a nurse, I have not physically laid down my life for a patient. On many occasions, I have experienced physical fatigue, and maybe even some minor emotional fatigue. However, through the continual pursuance of the great love of which Jesus spoke, I have been able to combat the spiritual battle of compassion fatigue. All praise be to God!

My Prayer for You

Heavenly Father,

Thank You for Jesus and the incredible free gift of salvation. Thank You for the illustration of the armor of God. This has provided protection for my heart, mind, and soul against compassion fatigue. I invite Your Holy Spirit to remain within me, so that I might continue to demonstrate unconditional, compassionate love to those entrusted in my care. I pray that the person reading this book will also invite You to live within their hearts, will obey Your commands, and love others fully and completely, and will serve their patients with a heart overflowing with compassion.

In Jesus' Holy and most precious name, Amen.

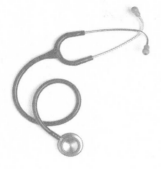

Chapter 22

Memorable Moments

Throughout this book you have read the many stories related to my personal experiences regarding nursing. You have experienced firsthand many of the patients for whom I have cared, how they impacted my life, and why nursing is a remarkably rewarding career. But I did not want you to only read and take my word for it. So I asked a few of my fellow nursing colleagues to put into their own words some of their most memorable nursing-career moments. This chapter is a compilation of their stories regarding the emotional, physical, and spiritual aspects of caring for patients and their families. It is my utmost honor and with deep appreciation that I include the stories of these admirable nurses in this book. I pray that their stories touch your heart as deeply as they have touched mine.

Temporary Home

Rebecca Hamon, MSN, RN

I began my nursing profession as a bedside nurse in the Neonatal Intensive Care Unit. I have always had such a passion for infants and believed that they are a blessing from our Heavenly Father! I felt so honored to care for infants who were born prematurely, sick, or battling other complications. I had experienced moments of intense joy and moments of pure sadness. It was a night I would forever remember as I walked onto the unit. I was informed that I would be caring for an infant who was diagnosed with anencephaly. Anencephaly is a neural tube defect that causes abnormal development of the brain and bones of the skull. Anencephaly is not compatible with life. The infant's parents were informed that they may only have a few minutes to a few hours with their son, Max.

As I processed the magnitude of loss that was about to occur, I prayed the Lord would equip me for the situation. The verse that came to my mind was Philippians 4:13, "I can do all things through Christ who strengthens me" (NKJV). I could not fathom carrying my child for nine months only to lose him in a matter of minutes or hours. However, I knew my God was sovereign and He does not give us more than we can handle. He knows our needs, hears our cries, and answers according to His will. You see, Max was not the only child that was soon to deliver. He had shared his home for the last nine months with his twin sister. I believe the Lord knew that this family would need another child to help cope with the loss of their son.

As the delivery process began, we were all prepared for what was to about to occur. Within a matter of minutes, a beautiful baby boy was born, but I couldn't help but notice that Max began to immediately fight for his life. I prayed, "Oh Lord, please don't let him go yet." After oxygen therapy was initiated, I placed Max on his mother's chest. He immediately began to turn pink and appeared in no distress! It was absolutely amazing! I was once again in awe of God's mercies.

Max continued to fight for his life for the next 24 hours before the Lord called him home. In that time, we were able to capture pictures with his twin sister, record his first bath on video, and create many memories that will last a lifetime. As heart wrenching as it was to watch his family say goodbye, I was forever grateful for the precious time that the Lord provided this family. As I mustered enough courage to walk down to the morgue and let Max go, I was reminded that this earth was just his temporary home. He was now in the arms of Jesus where he will live eternally. I look forward to the day when I will not only see my Heavenly Father, but will once again be reunited with sweet baby Max.

Discrete Dignity

Kristin Jaye Henderson, MSN, RN

I loved being a pediatric nurse. I had the privilege of working with patients from a couple weeks old through adolescence. One of the greatest honors of being a nurse is maintaining patient dignity. As nurses we see patients when they are the most vulnerable and fragile. Sometimes the greatest gift we can give is to see past this current state they are in and make them feel whole again. In reflecting back on a memorable moment in my career, I think of an adolescent female patient, B, that I cared for. This patient had major bowel surgery and had a very painful and long recovery. Thankfully, she asked for me to be her primary nurse, so I got to be a part of her healing process. This patient was very much a typical teenage girl. She liked makeup, dressing up, and certainly liked boys. One day I helped her put on her prettiest purple robe, made sure her hair looked nice, and took her to the teen room. It was so wonderful to see her smile and talk with other patients her age. It seemed as if she had forgotten all about her pain. B was having such a good time, she didn't notice the fecal leakage she left behind in her chair. I very discreetly covered it with a towel and returned later to clean the soiled area with an antibacterial cleanser. No one even knew it ever happened. I don't even think B knew that I did this for her. The satisfaction of maintaining her dignity was enough for me.

It's the Small Things

Bonnie Todd, MSN, APRN, FNP-BC

In my 35 years of nursing, I have been blessed with many memorable encounters with many wonderful patients. One such an encounter stands out in my mind.

A young father of three was to be seen at 9:00 that morning in follow-up for his multiple sclerosis. He was well known to me, having treated him for the last five years. Mentally reviewing the last few months with his setbacks and many complications, his voiced concerns came back to me with the emotional impact and compassion experienced at that time. He wanted to be able to continue to work and support his family, be a husband to his wife, and be able to afford his $2,000.00/month medications. This amazing young man of strong character and faith was not complaining, but wanting to aggressively address these issues.

We had spent the better part of the last two visits tackling these issues. His medications were reviewed and letters to the pharmaceutical companies were written. A vigorous physical therapy plan was discussed and orders written for implementation. The more delicate issues of intimacy were also addressed with recommendations for both he and his wife to have counseling. We discussed the potential problems related to his work environment. An appointment was made with a work specialist in kinesiology to better adapt his environment to his special needs. The visit ended with prayer and Scriptures that were written down for further review and study.

As I continued to consider, it didn't really seem that I had done a great deal; no magic drugs, no pat answers, no promises of recovery, and no guarantees that this disease could or would be contained. What would today's visit bring? What more could be offered?

The staff announced he had arrived and was waiting in the exam room. Offering a prayer for wisdom, I went down the hall to greet him. I was totally taken back. His youngest daughter was with him. She had a tree with hand-painted eggs on a red, heart-shaped platform. She said she and her daddy had made this for me to say thank you for taking such good care of her daddy. Tears welled up in my eyes as I hugged both of them.

This encounter was ten years ago. I still have the "egg tree" on my shelf in my kitchen so that I remember to pray for that patient and his beautiful family. What seemed so little in my eyes was very significant in their eyes. Compassionate care is sometimes just listening and filling out papers, with His love!

The Important Things in Life

Dr. Linda Moran, PhD, RN

The steps of a man are established by the LORD, when he delights in his way (Psalm 37:23).

God orders our steps and teaches us throughout our lives. With me, God chose to do just that when, in the prime of my nursing career, I was given the opportunity for employment as a hospice, on-call nurse.

A hospice nurse was not what I expected to be, and I wondered about the key lessons that would be important in life as I observed dying people at the end of their life. I wondered, "Why this and why now?" Over the course of the five years I spent in hospice nursing, God answered my questions by repeatedly showing me not the why, but the what — "what is important in life."

I didn't have to wonder too long, as I was able to clearly see the answer within a few months of practice. Every hospice patient for whom I cared taught me something different. One woman of my same age who had end-stage lung cancer said to me, "Lighten up, I intend to live every one of these final days to the fullest and, if you are going to be my nurse, you need to do that with me."

Regardless of the beliefs the patient had about life, being surrounded by people who loved them was the one request they had: to have loved ones present with them as they walked each step of their unique dying journey. Many did not know how to die and they asked me several times, "How do I die? I've never done this before." Although skilled at the effective management of pain, I soon realized that management of pain and mental suffering is a far more effective tool when coupled with the application of gentle compassion. Born-again Christians were not afraid of where they were going after death, but the actual dying process was frightening and unfamiliar to them. They knew their Savior was waiting for them with open arms, nevertheless, they had times when they wondered why their bodies were feeling so different and painful and unlike anything they had ever experienced. Knowing Jesus as my Savior was the precious prayer and conversation connection that helped them bridge this frightening experience.

After many months of watching the gathering, the loving, the pain, the fear, and the release, I learned the balm that made it all better to some degree was the compassionate touch, nearness, and presence of not only their loved ones but of those administering hospice care to them. The gathering of their loved ones loving on them was a process that sometimes even delayed their final breath. They taught me that life and death were about the same things: it was not about the amount of money in the bank or the diplomas on the wall or all their life's accomplishments.

Rather, easing the dying process was about forgiveness and love, it was about tying up loose ends and making their peace before they left and crossed over to be with the Lord.

A Difficult Lesson

Dana Rookstool, MSN, RN

Nursing does not separate itself from the nurse when stepping off the unit, out of the office, or by exiting the university campus. Nursing becomes an inseparable identity, imprinted with a unique calling and deliberate commitment to serve others. I am a nurse (humbly spoken) therefore I can . . . make a difference.

We have unique opportunities to be that nurse making the difference as we intersect with people in a variety of circumstances. Our opportunities often find our patients in some of their most vulnerable moments — some happy, but many times very challenging or sad. I found that early in my career I was most comfortable in critical care. Here I could intervene and usually see an immediate response in the way of improved values on the telemetry monitors or physical assessment. I could titrate intravenous fluids and vasoactive drugs to regulate blood pressure and improve my patients' heart rate and urine output. I was always proud to see our patients "graduate" to the step-down unit, which indicated that they successfully crossed the great divide between their critical state and a healing journey. One last pep talk and they were on their way . . . rarely did I ever see them again.

Since "the early days" of my nursing career, God has graciously revealed to me the larger picture. The years in critical care were an essential contrast for me to have alongside a world on the other side of the curtain — outside of the sterile, technical, controlled setting where a script could be followed and resources were many. You see, a nurse is *the* nurse on whatever ground his/her feet occupy. Whether it is a school, church, the grocery store, an airplane, or anywhere in between, everyone expects the nurse they know to be *on call*. If your identity is unknown to others, it is inescapable to self. It is that permeation of who we are that innately drives us to be available for others in need — but, in need of what?

Oh, the places we'll follow . . . our (adult) children. We journeyed via planes, trains, and autos to Bhopal, India, where our daughter and her husband were working with young couples in missionary work. On one very rainy, humid afternoon I felt drawn to one of their university hospitals, where I coerced our clan to try to gain a tour of their pediatric unit.

Our distinctly American presence attracted reluctant and armed security guards outside the main entrance who eventually granted us supervised entrance. Although I did not expect a contemporary setting, I was still ill-prepared to see the over-crowded, undersized, ward-style, resource-less area that housed ill children and their families on cots, mats, and in cribs. As the doors swung shut behind me, I could no longer be just an observer. Several sets of troubled eyes looked my way. It was strangely quiet with infrequent infant cries. One mother sat with her tiny infant on the floor in an isolated area with no furniture. The 20-year-old, soft-spoken nurse, caring for the needs of the entire unit, explained in broken English the sadness of this premature, failure-to-thrive infant.

At the end of the ward, in what looked like a makeshift critical care area, a preschooler was battling malaria. A ventilator was breathing for him; his emaciated suite-mate had typhoid. So many needs, and what could I offer? After a few smiles, nods, and attempting to encourage the Indian nurse called to the middle of this battle zone, I left feeling that I should have been prepared to do more.

Later, a young man who appeared to have suffered the effects of polio was ambulating along on his knuckles and one knee, sentenced to a life of begging. He said nothing, but presented himself at our feet with his hand out as we prepared to board our auto. Warned not to give money, as it typically falls into the hands of others, we regrettably avoided the uncomfortable pause and stepped toward our ride, leaving him void of rupees while I avoided that still small voice — *what is the message on his heart?*

These images will eternally haunt me. It is difficult to *not* notice those seemingly "discarded" in places like India on the street and in the hospitals, but those *feeling* discarded and without hope are everywhere. The technical training I had as a nurse failed me in my unpreparedness. The bigger lesson, however, for me was being fully present in the moment to' more fully understand the "in need of what" that I can extend without physical resources — actively valuing another human being. This is simply done through intentional eye contact, holding a hand, and reaching beyond barriers to communicate each one's worth and value as created by God with a purpose. Each is uniquely known by our Creator, who knows and understands all details of our lives:

> Are not two sparrows sold for a penny? Yet not one of them will fall to the ground outside your Father's care. And even the very hairs of your head are all numbered. So don't be afraid; you are worth more than many sparrows (Matthew 10:29–31; NIV).

My plan is to return to India. The opportunities with those that I sidestepped before may not be retrieved, but God's mercies are new each day. Wherever we are, there are always those in need of spiritual truth and the understanding that they are valued by our Heavenly Father. How we communicate this on an elementary level is typically universal — to notice and deliberately make a genuine effort to do so should be as integrated into our very being as nursing is to the nurse. What a privilege we have to do so!

> A new command I give you: Love one another. As I have loved you, so you must love one another. By this everyone will know that you are my disciples, if you love one another (John 13:34–35; NIV).

Divine Appointment

Karen Shepherd, MSN, RN, CHSE

As I walked into room 210 to complete my oncoming shift assessments, I noticed the patient in bed 2 was uneasy. His diagnosis was Chronic Obstructive Pulmonary Disease (COPD) and he was stable. Yet despite a normal assessment and breathing effortlessly, something was wrong. As I questioned him, he stated he was scared because he knew he was going to die. I secretly doubted his feelings, but I knew he was frightened and I had the answer to take away his anxiety.

I had only been a graduate nurse for six weeks. I was not overly confident and was unsure of hospital policies concerning spiritual issues. Would I get in trouble for sharing my faith and telling him about Jesus? I decided it didn't matter — he needed peace that only Jesus could provide.

I had never shared my faith with a patient. I felt very inadequate explaining how he could have assurance that he was going to heaven if he died. To my surprise, he said he wanted to accept Jesus as his personal Savior. We prayed together, he confessed his sin and believed Jesus was his Savior. I saw a change in his face after we prayed. I could see peace and relief. I left his room and he slept peacefully the entire night.

Two nights later when I returned to work, I was anxious to see the patient in room 210, bed 2. I noticed his name was not on the census board. I asked the staff about him and, to my astonishment, they said he had died the day before. I was shocked and thankful. This man knew he was leaving this earth and I didn't believe him; however, I was thankful that God had used me to tell this man about God's love and salvation, and he had accepted. I look forward to meeting this man in heaven someday.

My Prayer for You

Heavenly Father,

I praise You for all of these extraordinary nurses. Thank You for instilling in them the passion and compassion that it takes to selflessly give of themselves and provide care to those in need. Thank You for creating us all with different desires, so that we can dedicate our lives to various aspects of nursing. The profession would not be so successful, valued, and respected if we all practiced in the same department, in the same fashion. Thank You for each of the memorable moments presented in this chapter. I pray that the person reading this book will recognize his or her value and will stop to savor the memorable moments that I am positive they will soon encounter if they enter this incredible profession called nursing.

In Jesus' Holy and most precious name, Amen.

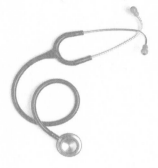

Chapter 23

Answering
the Call

"Only let each person lead the life that the Lord has assigned to him, and to which God has called him" (1 Corinthians 7:17), and "Whatever you do, do all to the glory of God" (1 Corinthians 10:31). The thought of leading a life in pursuit of the fulfillment of the calling assigned to one by God and doing all things for the glory of God may seem both daunting and exhilarating. However, let me assure you that God has placed a calling on all whom He created. Since God is the creator of heaven, the earth, and everything that inhabits the earth, that means he created you; and you, assuredly, possess a calling upon your life that is awaiting fulfillment. The questions remaining are, "What is your calling?" and "How shall you answer it?"

Prayerfully, you have been pondering these questions as you have read this book. Each chapter journeyed you deeper into the sanctity and sacredness of a career within the profession of nursing. You were introduced to some of the history of nursing; explored the purpose of a nurse; dispelled some of the myths associated with the profession; peered into the lives of patients;

uncovered key attributes required of a nurse of excellence; examined curriculum choices, varying degrees, salaries, and the endless opportunities associated with nursing; journeyed through some of the hardships encountered working in the profession; and learned how to persevere and remain nourished while fulfilling such an incredible calling.

Now, it is up to you! The first step in answering a call is intently listening. "To answer before listening — that is folly and shame" (Proverbs 18:13; NIV). You must listen to the still, small voice of the Holy Spirit within you, discerning whether or not your heart is being beckoned to this rewarding profession. I am not claiming that God is going to show up in your living room and provide you with your life's play-by-play, but if it is His will for your life, He will quicken your spirit and place a burning desire within you for helping and serving others through nursing. "'For I know the plans I have for you,' declares the LORD, 'plans to prosper you and not to harm you, plans to give you hope and a future'" (Jeremiah 29:11; NIV). You may never feel that you have a black and white, cut-and-dry answer as to whether or not nursing is your calling, but you can rest in knowing that God does have great plans for your life.

After all, He created you, knitted you together in your mother's womb, blessed you with a unique personality, and placed distinct desires within your heart. Just like fingerprints and snowflakes, every human being was designed to be different. Although we are all members of the Body of Christ, "if the whole body were an eye, where would be the sense of hearing? If the whole body were an ear, where would be the sense of smell?" (1 Corinthians 12:17). Likewise, if every person was a nurse, where would be the lawyer, teacher, factory worker, or chef? Our society would not function very well if we were all nurses. Thus, "God arranged the members in the body, each one of them, as he chose" (1 Corinthians 12:18).

As you are journeying throughout life, attempting to figure out where your place is within this arrangement, be sure to pay close attention to the small things. Does your heart skip a beat at the thought of saving a life? Do you experience a feeling of satisfaction when you help someone solve a problem? Or has anyone (like my call to nursing) ever told you that you would make a great nurse? These may seem like subtle experiences. However, they may be the Holy Spirit attempting to get your attention. The key is to be still and listen. God speaks to us through His Holy Scripture (the Bible), through our experiences, and through the words of other people.

So if you feel that may be hearing a call to the profession of nursing, but are still in the gray area regarding nursing as a career, I challenge you to go ahead and start exploring nursing programs at various colleges and universities. Write down ten of the most important qualities that you need in order to experience joy while attending school. If one of your requirements is quality time with family, maybe a college close to home would work best for you. If you possess the desire and anticipation of acceptance into an advanced practice nursing program, perhaps it would be advisable to find a college or university that is ranked among some of the nation's elite. If affordability is high on your list, searching for a college with tuition meeting your budget requirements is vital. No matter what comprises your "list," it is imperative that you do not forget that the most important aspect of a nursing career is the people entrusted to your care. If you discover a program that meets every quality on your list, but does not value people, then I encourage you to continue seeking. Do not accept mediocrity when it comes to the importance placed on human life.

You may never find a nursing program that meets all ten qualifications on your list. But I urge you to pay close attention to the program's mission, vision, and philosophy. If these are in direct opposition with your values and beliefs, then it is probably not the place for you. Furthermore, pay close attention to the program's accreditation status and NCLEX pass rates. These are two important aspects that potentially indicate the quality of a nursing program's curriculum and instruction.

Once you have discovered the nursing program that meets many or all of your qualifications, it is time to ensure that you meet the qualifications of the program. Most nursing programs will have a document delineating potential applicant qualifications listed on their website. Peruse this list and ensure that you meet the criteria. If you do not fully understand the qualifications, do not be afraid to pick up the phone and contact the nursing department's manager. These individuals possess a wealth of information and can usually walk you through each step necessary to complete the application process.

However, please do not have your heart set on one program. You should create a rank-order list of at least three programs in which you are interested and could apply. Nursing programs can be extremely competitive and you do not want to miss out on your calling because you did not get into your first-choice program. Remember, "The heart of man plans his way, but the LORD establishes his steps" (Proverbs 16:9).

Furthermore, "Do not be anxious about anything, but in everything by prayer and supplication with thanksgiving let your requests be made known to God" (Philippians 4:6). This is our instruction to pray. Listening and praying are requirements in order to truly recognize, realize, and answer any call placed upon your life. Do not worry or fret about all of the details. Simply take one step at a time. Anxiety and worry will merely slow you down and do not catalyze the process in any way. I love the Scripture: "And which of you by being anxious can add a single hour to his span of life?" (Luke 12:25). How true! So, slow down, take a deep breath, pray, listen, and prepare your heart for the most sacred journey which you will ever take . . . answering and fulfilling the call to nursing.

My Prayer for You

Heavenly Father,

First of all, I want to thank You so much for your unconditional love. Thank You for calling me to be a nurse, and for continually renewing my passion, compassion, and love for people. Thank You for allowing me to share my heart through this book. I pray that it will deeply touch the hearts and lives of every reader. Father, You created each one of us with unique ambitions and desires. Please provide each reader with a spirit of discernment. Open their eyes and ears to see and hear all that You have for them in this life. May they be able to truly be still and listen. Help them to be obedient and trust the plans that You have for them. Decrease any anxieties or fears that they may possess regarding their future. Father, make the path along the journey to answering their call, straight. I praise You and thank You for each and every person reading this book and pray that You bless them beyond measure, as You have daily blessed me.

In Jesus' Holy and most precious name, Amen.